Making Health Policy

Making Health Policy

A Critical Introduction

Andy Alaszewski and
Patrick Brown

polity

First published in 2012 by Polity Press

Polity Press
65 Bridge Street
Cambridge CB2 1UR, UK

Polity Press
350 Main Street
Malden, MA 02148, USA

ISBN-13: 978-0-7456-4173-7
ISBN-13: 978-0-7456-4174-4(pb)

A catalogue record for this book is available from the British Library.

Typeset in 10.5 on 12 pt Plantin
by Servis Filmsetting Ltd, Stockport, Cheshire
Printed and bound in Great Britain by MPG Books Group Limited, Bodmin, Cornwall

For further information on Polity, visit our website: www.politybooks.com

Contents

Preface

This text has been in gestation for over thirty years. In the early 1980s I was working in the Institute of Health Studies at the University of Hull and had the opportunity to write a critique of health policy making in the 1970s based on the Institute's programme of research (Haywood and Alaszewski 1980). At the time there were no textbooks dealing with the overall development of health policy and therefore I made a proposal to a major publisher's series editor for such a textbook. For reasons that are not entirely clear to me the proposal was not accepted and for me it was a missed opportunity.

I was therefore delighted when Polity Press approached me and invited me to write a textbook on health policy making. I now had a young colleague at the University of Kent, Patrick Brown, who taught policy-making modules with me and who could contribute to the writing. My own ideas had developed considerably. The book I planned to write in the 1980s would have been heavily influenced and shaped by British social and public administration, especially the work of Ron Brown, with whom I worked in Hull, and Frank Stacey, whose work I admired. It would have had a very strong historical structure focusing on the evolution and development of health policy making. I remain interested in this aspect of health policy making and in this book we draw both on historical material and on political sciences, but since successive editions of excellent textbooks by Rudolf Klein (2001) and Chris Ham (2004) cover this aspect, it is not as prominent in this book as it was in my original proposal.

In the past twenty years I have become increasingly interested in the broader social and psychological processes underlying policy making, and these interests have been reinforced through the collaboration with Patrick Brown and, as a result, this text focuses on a major tension and contradiction in the policy process. We were interested in the need for policy makers to present and justify their policies as rational – i.e. the best, most effective and beneficial response to particular issues – while at the same time managing the realities and irrationalities of everyday life such as the emotional consequences of disasters or the pressure of a critical tabloid press.

Our approach to policy making is shaped by our interest in the ways in which risk is constructed and managed in contemporary society. We are both involved in risk research and publishing as editor and deputy editor of the international journal *Health, Risk and Society*. There are important similarities between risk management and policy making. Both processes form part of the Enlightenment programme of managing present uncertainties and creating better futures by using scientific knowledge developed through the empirical study of past events. Both risk managers and policy makers would like to see themselves as objective experts who identify the best and most rational solutions to the threats and problems facing society, and both face the difficulties of communicating the benefits of their proposed solutions, especially to groups to individuals who do not share their perceptions and knowledge, i.e. who adopt a less rational approach.

Some issues we explore in this book are actually more clearly articulated in risk studies. The different perceptions and influences of those at the core of policy making and the wider society need to be teased out by considering the limitations imposed on core policy makers by events such as disasters or pressure from the mass media. In risk studies the difference between 'expert' understanding and management of risk and those of lay people is a central theme. Expert risk managers focus on the 'objective' measurement of hazards and use structured decision-making systems to predict and manage the future. From their perspective lay responses are irrational and need to be changed through the effective communication of risk. Individuals living in a complex world do not have the time, resources or inclinations to use time-consuming and complex processes based on technical rationality but instead tend to rely on 'short cuts' such as 'common sense', their emotions or trust, which usually work effectively (Alaszewski and Brown 2007; Alaszewski and Coxon 2008).

In both policy and risk studies, a narrow focus on key decision makers emphasises the technical aspects of the process and in particular how these decision makers access and use knowledge to inform their decisions. Risk managers and policy makers start from the position that objective measurable challenges exist and their job is to use reason and rationality to understand the nature of such challenges and to identify actions. Broadening the perspective shifts the focus to issues of framing, especially the ways in which some issues get defined as worthy of attention at a particular time whereas others equally or more challenging do not. Thus, in the context of risk, researchers have explored why, out of the myriad of potential threats facing an individual or social group, some are taken seriously and treated as risks whereas others are disregarded. In the context of policy, a similar interest is evident in studies of claims making and why core policy makers are receptive to some claims about social problems but not others. (We explore these issues more fully in chapter 6, and for a fuller discussion of these issues see Heyman et al. 2010.)

Our family, friends and colleagues have supported and contributed to this book. I would like to thank Helen Alaszewski for her continuing confidence, which has helped me through some difficult challenges in recent years, and it has been a great pleasure collaborating with her on research projects. Kirstie Coxon contributed to early discussions of the book. Adam Burgess worked with me on an editorial on risk, disasters and inquiries that influenced my thinking on chapter 5 (Alaszewski and Burgess 2007). Bob Heyman has been a close collaborator on risk and his ideas have influenced this book; and he was kind enough to read and comment on a pre-publication draft.

We both contributed to the overall development of this book and share responsibility for its content. However, I took the lead in writing chapters 1–5, 9 and 10, Patrick took the lead on chapters 6 to 8.

Andy Alaszewski

Introduction

This book focuses on the nature of health policy making in the United Kingdom. In the first part of the book we examine the importance of rationality in policy making and the ways in which core policy makers try to make their policies rational. We start by looking inside the policy process, considering the factors that shape the rationality of health policy. We start chapter 1 with a discussion of the modern conception of policy and its grounding in the Enlightenment concept of human progress and modernisation. We argue that in modern democracies policy makers need to justify their policies in terms of instrumental rationality: the measurable benefits which their policies have for citizens and the ways in which their policies will create a better future for all citizens. We consider the implications of this for health. We note that, in the United Kingdom, health is a relatively recent area of government interest, and policy making. Premodern governments lacked both the technology to improve health and an overall interest in the health of the population. In the nineteenth and early twentieth century, developments in public health and medicine provided the means for increased state intervention, and the development of social democracies with their commitment to enhancing the welfare of their citizens provided the stimulus and rationale for government involvement in health care, making health a major policy area. The formation of the NHS in 1948 can be seen as part of the 'Enlightenment' programme in which government has taken on responsibility for an important aspect of the welfare of its citizens and, as such, can be seen as both rational and progressive. However, we show through a discussion of the changing focus of health policy since 1948 that there have been major changes in focus, and what is considered rational has changed, reflecting the specific circumstances of the time.

In chapter 2 we start to explore how core policy makers – ministers and their advisers – seek to make policy making rational through using knowledge about the nature of health issues and the best way of addressing them. We start with the major paradox of policy making in the UK system, ministers' knowledge deficit. Ministers are senior and usually skilful politicians but they are not expected to have special interest in or knowledge of the policies for which they are given responsibility. They overcome this deficit through the use of confidential advisers, special political advisers and civil servants. The ways in which these advisers support the making of rational policy and the continual pressure to increase access to knowledge can be seen in and through the development of ministries that support health and related policy making.

In chapter 3 we concentrate on a key aspect of policy making and one which should reflect and facilitate rationality, the allocation of resources – particularly money – to health and related programmes. Money is concrete, objective and measurable and therefore is an ideal medium for thinking about the means/ends relationship that underpins instrumental rationality. However, as we will show, the complexity of predicting the changes in the cost of programmes and changes in prices means that it is impossible to achieve rationality, which would require a review of all past decisions. There is rationality in public expenditure decisions but it is very much in the margins of overall allocations, in the decisions about which policies will receive additional or reduced funding. There are the practical limitations to full rationality – especially the limitations of time, knowledge and resources – and the pressure of external events, and core policy makers deal with these limitations by making decisions which are good enough in the circumstances, although not the best.

In chapter 4 we explore the ways in which core policy makers – Ministers and their civil servants – draw on external expertise through policy communities and networks. We examine the ways in which policy communities provide core policy makers with a cost-effective way of overcoming some of the practical problems of accessing knowledge. By building up trustworthy relationships with a range of individuals and groups with expertise in particular aspects of policy, core policy makers – especially civil servants – can expand the quantity and quality of knowledge which informs decision making. In health policy making, such trusted groups have traditionally included those closely involved in the provision of health care, such as health professionals, health authorities and drug companies. However, other groups also have expertise, for example those representing alternative practitioners or particular groups of health service users. These groups are often not perceived as trustworthy and their knowledge and beliefs may challenge those of the insider core of policy makers. Thus these outsider groups may be perceived as a threat and only involved in the policy process when there is no alternative. We note in chapter 4 that there has been a major change in the ways in which core policy makers interact with other groups. During the early period of the NHS, there was a club culture in which medical groups such as the British Medical Association (BMA) were co-opted into health policy making. As the scale, complexity and cost of health and related care increased so did the range of groups consulted. The BMA lost its privileged insider status as core policy makers moved to a more open system of consultation with an emphasis on involving patients and the public in all aspects of decision making.

In chapter 5 we move on to consider the pressure of events, especially disasters, on health policy making. Rational policy making needs time and resources for the dispassionate analysis of issues and the selection of the best policies to address them. Events such as disasters reduce the scope of rational action. They often create an emotionally charged atmosphere in which there is pressure for immediate action by core policy makers. Ministers can buy time by appointing independent inquiries but only at the cost of acknowledging that routine policy making has failed and the risk that the inquiry will recommend unacceptable policy changes. We examine the increasing importance of disasters in health and social care policy making. We note the ways in which, in the immediate postwar period, the NHS and related services were protected and, while major service failure could result in serious harm to service users and others, this harm tended to remain a private misfortune and did not become a public disaster. However, for a variety of reasons, this protection was reduced, and disasters and associated inquiries have become almost a routine part of policy making.

In the second part of the book we shift the focus of attention from the policy making process and the core policy makers to a broader societal context. This involves a move beyond rationality – i.e. the view that objective knowledge about health problems and their solutions exists independently of policy makers – to a more socially grounded perspective that acknowledges and examines the political and social processes that structure knowledge of health and related problems and their solutions. Indeed, we reconsider several of the cases from Part 1 using this perspective. Since these processes are interconnected, the structure of the second part of the book is to some extent arbitrary and the themes overlap. Thus, when we deal with the processes of claims making in 'creating' social problems (chapter 6), we acknowledge that the openness of social democracies facilitates the articulation of competitive claims (chapter 7), that ideologies contribute to the definition or framing of such claims (chapter 8) and that the media provide a major forum for the articulation of claims (chapter 9).

While in chapter 5 we emphasise the way in which an apparently rational bureaucratic formalism can be disrupted and ruptured by disasters and unforeseen events, chapter 6 goes on to peer into the processes by which seemingly obvious concerns for policy makers are made into 'problems'. We draw upon claims-making and constructionist approaches to policy – to develop an account of how interested parties are involved in bringing certain issues to the attention of policy makers, as well as reasons why certain claims-makers and their claims are more successful than others. Here, notions of power become strongly evident in terms of the mechanisms by which certain interests are able to influence policy-making while other significant interests and social conditions remain 'unarticulated'. Amidst this tension between competing interests, policy-making comes to be seen more as a disjointed amalgam of conflicting notions.

In chapter 7 we develop a broader understanding of the context of this claims-making and, more particularly, the nature of health policy within a modern democracy. Both the nature of democratic accountability and, moreover, the way this format manifests itself within late-modern environments have implications for how policy makers reach policy decisions and justify these to a diverse audience. The pragmatic policy formats which emerge in this context raise important questions regarding whether the influence of the public in the complex and highly technical business of running health-care systems is a positive or negative phenomenon. We also draw attention to various ways in which suspicions regarding a democratic deficit have been addressed and the tensions that emerge within such schemes of public involvement.

Underlying the features covered in the first two chapters of part 2 of the book is a deeper notion of ideology. In chapter 8 we make this multifaceted and often nebulous concept more explicit – specifically addressing the role of ideology and its use in legitimating policies across diverse groups, necessarily bounding what policy makers are concerned with, and the corresponding way health issues are framed in certain terms and in relation to certain actors. Ideology, as a way of linking policy and health-care activities to particular values, is explored at a number of different levels. Dominant societal discourses and knowledge paradigms are implicit in the assumptions policy makers bring to their work, while ideologies are also invoked more explicitly to win support and make sense of the contexts of which policy is product.

Underlying many of the phenomena which we discuss in the second part of this book is one of the most important institutions of modern society, the mass media. The media are the major source of knowledge about events and activities which individuals, including core policy makers, cannot experience for themselves. They provide the main forum in which claims-makers make their claims. They are one of the key elements of an open democratic society and they are the place in which modern ideologies are articulated. The mass media are not neutral or passive. Their elements, such as newspapers, play an active role in selecting information and promoting interest, claims and ideologies. Thus in modern society core policy makers have to react to the agenda being set by the mass media and often have to make rapid decisions in order to avoid blame in emotionally charged situations.

In the concluding chapter we note that for policy makers the gap between the ideals and realities of policy making create a serious challenge, and they continually attempt to bridge this gap, often seeking technical solutions such as changes in the machinery of policy making or more and better knowledge. However, the reality for policy makers is that they have to operate within an environment that is increasingly unpredictable and uncontrollable and in which they try to demonstrate their ability to identify and control those factors that will create a better future while avoiding the blame for inevitable failures. For policy analysts, it is more interesting and fun. It is possible to identify some of the factors that influence policy outcomes. For example, it is possible to predict that participants in the policy process with veto power, the most resources, that are the most media savvy and have the best evidence to support their claims are likely to have the greatest influence on policy outcomes. However, the precise policy outcome depends on the unique circumstances of each case.

1

What is health policy?

AIMS

To consider the ways in which modern government and policy making have developed, the influence of Enlightenment thinking on the purposes of government and policy making, and the increasing importance of health as an area of policy making.

OBJECTIVES

- To consider the ways in which the role of government and the nature of policy have changed and the need for modern policy makers to justify their policies in terms of benefits to the population
- To examine how in social democracies with their commitment to enhancing the welfare of their citizens, government involvement in the provision of health care has increased and health has become a major policy area
- To review the ways in which health policy has changed since the formation of the NHS in 1948.

In this opening chapter we consider the definition and nature of government and health policy. We start by considering the modern conception of policy and its grounding in the Enlightenment concept of human progress and modernisation. This approach reflects the belief that it is possible to predict and improve the future through the rational application of knowledge. Within health, this involves the rational planning of health services to minimise disease and suffering. Given the expansion of scientific knowledge on the nature and causes of disease, this approach to health policy making emphasises the importance of technical expertise in defining health problems and in identifying, evaluating and adopting the most effective approaches to dealing with such problems.

1.1 The development of modern policy making: the importance of rationality

Policy making as the core government function

As with many important concepts, policy and policy making are often assumed to be self-evident. For example Ham and Hill (1993) in their policy textbook avoid defining policy by talking about policy analysis, citing Dye's definition:

> Policy analysis is finding out what governments do, why they do it, and what difference it makes. (Dye 1976 cited in Ham and Hill 1993: 4)

Given the difficulties in defining policy and policy making, some commentators just treat them as part of the overall process of government or governance. For example, Richards and Smith define governance as 'a descriptive label that is used to highlight the changing nature of policy process in recent decades. In particular, it sensitizes us to the ever-increasing variety of terrains and actors involved in the making of public policy. Thus, governance demands that we consider all actors and locations beyond the "core executive" involved in the policy-making process' (Richards and Smith 2002: 15).

Though it is clear that policy making is something that governments do, it is important to understand what it is and why they do it, and to understand this we explore the evolution of modern government and in particular the impact of the Enlightenment on the nature of government and policy making.

Influence of the Enlightenment on government and policy making

While government in the United Kingdom has evolved over a millennium, the origins of contemporary policy making are more recent and can be traced back to the eighteenth-century Enlightenment.

Prior to the eighteenth century, governments tended to focus on a

---

Box 1.1   The Enlightenment, government and policy making

The Enlightenment and modernity The eighteenth-century Enlightenment can be seen as an intellectual assault on traditional institutions, especially in France. It drew inspiration from the development of the scientific method in natural sciences and sought to apply the same methods, with the same benefits, to society and social relations. It was underpinned by a commitment to social progress and modernisation of institutions through radical change or revolution.

Implications for government Enlightenment thinkers attacked political institutions such as the absolute monarchy, and especially the religious legitimation of the French *Ancien Régime* based on the monarch's claim to Divine Right. They sought to create new rational political systems based on agreement or a Social Contract between citizens and their government. In this contract the government agreed to govern with the consent of and in the interests of citizens. For example, the American colonists justified their revolution and rebellion against the British monarch, George III, in a Declaration of Independence by the thirteen United States (1776) that stated that: 'We hold these truths to be self-evident, that all men are created equal, that they are endowed by their Creator with certain unalienable Rights, that among these are Life, Liberty and the pursuit of Happiness. — That to secure these rights, Governments are instituted among Men, deriving their just powers from the consent of the governed . . . ' (ushistory n.d.).

Implications for policy making In rational Enlightenment political systems, government actions and policy making can no longer be justified in terms of the greater glory of monarchs or the execution of God's Will but have to be justified in terms of the benefits that such actions and policies have for citizens. Philosophers such as Jeremy Bentham sought to create a rational basis for such administration by creating a system for measuring the benefits or happiness created by government so that leaders could demonstrate to citizens that their policies were ensuring the maximum benefit or greatest happiness of the greatest number.

limited range of activities and respond to problems in ad hoc fashion. If a problem arose, then a practical solution was sought. When such a solution involved radical change it was usually legitimated as a re-statement of traditional customs and practices. As Holt notes, the most radical medieval statement of civil liberties in England, the Magna Carta of 1215, 'pretended to state customary law' (1992: 1). In England this pragmatic approach to policy was reflected by the importance of traditional customs codified in statutory and Common Law. Statutory law was produced on the occasions when monarchs summoned Parliament, the Lords and representatives of the Commons, to vote additional taxes to enable them to fight their wars. On such occasions Lords and other members of Parliament were able to voice their grievances, and the response to such griev-ances would take the form of an Act of Parliament or statute. Grievances could be individually raised with the king's judges, and the judges would 'restate' the customary principles that informed their judgements. These principles, shared by or common to differ-ent jurisdictions, formed Common Law, legitimated by 'immemorial Usage or Custom' (see Hale 1713).

Contemporary governments tend to see the world and their role in a very different way. They emphasise their roles as innovators seeking to manage a complex and changing environment. Thus their orienta-tion is not to the past; they do not use past custom and practice to legitimate their actions. They look to the future, emphasising the way in which their activities are innovative and reforming, and will improve the future for the whole of society. This signifies a major change in the value of action and intervention in society. Premodern governments saw themselves as functioning in an ordered world and therefore only needed to intervene in society if there were signs of disorder, such as rebellion or grievances, and then their actions were to re-establish the order. In contrast, post-Enlightenment governments see the world as imperfect and their role is to improve it. Thus their imperative is to act, to change and to intervene. As Moran (2003) has argued, this has resulted in a situation of hyperinnovation in the late twentieth century as each new government introduces its own interventions and reforms. For example, in England, following an initial period of stability in the structure of the NHS (1948–74), the NHS has continu-ally been restructured or, in Enlightenment terms, modernised, with major restructuring in 1974, 1990–5, 1997–2000, 2007–8 and possibly 2012.

While modern governments are aware of individual problems and grievances and, in exceptional circumstances, they may develop policies in response to specific individual problems (see chapter 5 for the role of specific events such as disasters and inquiries in the formation of policy), such grievances tend to be filtered out by various mechanisms such as complaints systems or by the judicial system, leaving government and its ministers to focus on the 'big picture', creating a better economic, political and social system that will benefit all citizens. Thus contemporary governments are essentially utopian in that they envisage an ideal world, such as the Welfare State in which all citizens are protected from the cradle to the grave, and then seek to create this ideal world. Contemporary policy making is about vision, the 'big idea' and creating change to achieve such vision. In its reflection on the nature of government in a policy statement on *Modernising Government* (Her Majesty's Government 1999), the UK government defined policy making as the process of translating vision into action: 'Policy making is the process by which governments translate their political vision into programmes and actions to deliver "outcomes" – desired changes in the real world' (Her Majesty's Government 1999: ch. 2 para. 1). The Department of Health also describes its policies in the following way: 'DH policies are designed to improve on existing arrangements in health and social care, and turn political vision into actions that should benefit staff, patients and the public' (Department of Health 2011a). Thus, policy making involves defining desirable ends, especially improvements in society, as well as evaluating and selecting the best means of achieving such ends.

The Prime Minister's Foreword to the *Modernising Government* White Paper repeatedly stressed his future-oriented vision:

> Modernising Government is a significant step forward in what is a long-term programme of reform. It puts in place a number of important initiatives, and sets out an agenda for the future. But in line with the Government's overall modernisation programme, in line with our policy of investment for reform, it is modernisation for a purpose: modernising government to get better government for a better Britain. (Blair 1998)

This definition of the role of government has its roots in the Enlightenment of the eighteenth century in which French intellectuals rejected traditional sources of authority such as the received wisdom of custom and religious belief. Drawing on the evidence of advances in science and technology, they argued that rational scientific methods should be applied to all aspects of human endeavour, including government. They envisaged creating an Encyclopaedia of all knowledge that could be used as a resource to create a new, improved, utopian social system. Their ideas influenced both the founding fathers of the United States, finding expression in its Constitution, and the revolutionaries who destroyed the *Ancien Régime* in France and tried to replace it with a rational system of government and social relations.

In Britain the influence of the Enlightenment on politics was less obvious. The conservative reaction to the various late eighteenth-century revolutions emphasised the uniqueness and robustness of British institutions and traditions, such as its unwritten constitution and its Common Law. This conservative reaction was linked to Romanticism, a movement evident in the arts and architecture that rejected the scientific rationality of the Enlightenment. For example, when the building that housed the British Parliament burnt down in 1834 the new building was not the favoured model of revolutionaries, a classic Greek revival structure with its democratic connotations, but a romanticised medieval structure emphasising the continuity of British traditions (Hill 2008). Romantics argued that rationality neglected and suppressed the essential nature of humanity – especially the emotional, religious and artistic expression of human experience (*Encyclopædia Britannica* 2010).

Utilitarianism and policy making

Despite the conservative reaction and the influence of Romanticism in Britain, Enlightenment ideas played a major role in reshaping government, especially through the ideas and work of utilitarians such as Jeremy Bentham and Edwin Chadwick and through reforms of the institutions, including Parliament and the civil service.

Bentham was committed to human progress and reform, especially to developing a rational basis for British law and legislation. In the Preface to 'A fragment on government', originally published in 1776, he noted that: 'The Age we live in is a busy age; in which knowledge is rapidly advancing towards perfection' (1977: ch. I para. 39). For Bentham the rational basis of government activity should be its utility, i.e. the extent to which such activity increased the 'benefit, advantage, pleasure, good or happiness' of the community (2000: ch. I para. III).

Bentham used the term 'utility' to refer to the positive effect of actions and he usually referred to these positive effects as 'happiness' and 'pleasure', contrasting them to negative effects such as pain. Though concepts such as 'happiness', 'pleasure' and 'pain' may seem

Box 1.2   QALYs: a means of measuring the utility of health care

Lack of a measure of impact of health   Although epidemiologists and government statisticians in the nineteenth century developed measures of the overall health of the population, such as life expectancy and the survival rates for specific diseases, there were in the 1960s no measures of the specific benefits of particular treatments. When the economist Alan Williams (1927–2005) was seconded to the Ministry of Health in the late 1960s he found that most of health policy making was evidence-free, with no systematic evaluation of the benefits of policies. A major problem was the lack of any way of measuring the impact of specific interventions.

Developing QALYs   When Williams returned to academic research at the University of York, he worked with colleagues to develop a measure of utility, the Quality Adjusted Life Year (QALY). This sought to measure the benefits of a particular treatment, such as a new drug for breast cancer, in terms of the additional number of years of life which a patient undergoing the treatment gained when compared to a patient not receiving treatment, adjusted and reduced to take into account any negative effects of the treatment such as pain or disability. Thus the QALY would represent the 'objective' benefits of the treatment, which could then form part of a cost–benefit analysis to assess the relative benefits of the treatment compared to non-treatment or the current standard form of treatment.

Using QALYs   QALYs are now routinely used by the National Institute of Health and Clinical Excellence (NICE) to evaluate the effectiveness of new drugs and treatments. NICE has discussed the criteria for its decision making, indicating that if a QALY costs less than £20,000, then the intervention is considered to be cost-effective. If a QALY costs between £20,000 and £30,000, then other factors should be considered, for example whether there are other substantial gains that have not been captured by this measure. If costs of a treatment are over £30,000, then the advisory body needs to make an even stronger case if it believes it should be funded (NICE 2008b: 19). These evaluations form the basis of NICE recommendations to health ministers about which new drugs and treatments should be adopted in and funded by the NHS (see chapter 2, box 2.8, and chapter 7, box 7.3, for two views of NICE recommendations relating to Herceptin, a treatment for breast cancer).

vague and subjective, Bentham argued that they could be objectively measured and therefore the utility or benefit of a particular action could and should be assessed. For Bentham the moral basis of all human actions was 'the production of the greatest possible quantity of happiness' (2000: ch. XVII para. II). A ruler should '*govern* the people in such a *particular* manner always as should be *subservient* to their happiness' (1977: ch. I para. 39, italics in the original), and therefore the moral basis for governing was the maximisation of the utility of all citizens: '*it is the greatest happiness of the greatest number that is the measure of right and wrong*' (Bentham 1977: Preface 393, italics in the original). Thus for Bentham the starting point for a rational system of policy making was a system for measuring the benefits of government actions and policies.

The economist Pareto subsequently refined Bentham's approach, arguing that the best course of action was one which made someone better off and did not make anyone worse off. Bentham wanted his ideas to be adopted to create a better society. For example, he was concerned with the relief of poverty and crime and made practical proposals for reforming the systems for dealing with these issues through such mechanisms as panopticons that would enable all prisoners or paupers to be observed and controlled from a central vantage point. His ideas influenced reformers (see box 1.4 for the New Poor Law).

While Britain avoided the major political convulsions and revolutions associated with the development of nation states in the nineteenth century, there was a major restructuring of government, albeit one spread over a longer period of time. The most visible aspects were the series of Reform Acts, starting in 1832 and culminating in 1921, that widened electoral participation from a narrow, propertied section of the male population to all adult men and women (see chapter 7 for further discussion). This move to 'mass' democracy stimulated the development of political parties, with their clearly articulated ideologies representing and mobilising defined interests with differentiated social bases. In turn, these political changes were associated with technological changes such as the development of the large-scale printing presses that facilitated the expansion of mass media that in turn influenced the nature of policy making (see chapter 9). A less visible but equally significant modification was the restructuring of the machinery of government (see chapter 2), with a clear differentiation between political or ministerial oversight of policy, expert policy advice provided by senior civil servants, and detailed operational management of government activity by junior civil servants.

The role of utilitarianism in contemporary government and policy making

Utilitarianism continues to have an important influence on the ways in which contemporary policy makers think about and justify their role. For example, Franklin D. Roosevelt, a radical reforming twentieth-century American President, echoed Bentham's words when he stated that: 'Always . . . your Government has had but one sign on its desk – 'Seek only the greater good of the greater number of Americans' (quoted in Dolbeare and Cummings 2004: 415).

Similarly in the White Paper that set out the blue-print for the post-war Welfare State in Britain, William Beveridge gave Bentham's formula a socialist slant:

> The object of government in peace and war is not the glory of rulers or of races but the happiness of the common man. (Beveridge 1942: pt 7)

In the United Kingdom, the government's review of current policy making, *Modernising Government* (Her Majesty's Government 1999) incorporated key elements of utilitarian philosophy. The review stated that policies 'should really deal with the problems', so creating benefits for citizens. The process of decision making should be rational, evidence-based and insulated from 'short-term pressures'. The outcomes should be measured 'by results rather than activity' (Her Majesty's Government 1999: ch. 2 para. 2). Given the increased emphasis on democracy since Bentham's time, the intended benefits of policy are not defined in terms of happiness but as 'delivering the outcomes people want' (Her Majesty's Government 1992: ch. 2 para. 1).

The changing nature of policy making: the case of the Poor Law

The changing nature of government activity and of policy making can be clearly seen by comparing responses to poverty in the sixteenth and nineteenth centuries (see boxes 1.3 and 1.4 which contrast the sixteenth-century Elizabethan and the nineteenth-century New Poor Laws). The Elizabethan Poor Laws can be seen as an incremental and ad hoc response to poverty. They were preceded by neither a thorough and expert review of the nature of the problem nor a systematic evaluation of the alternative ways of dealing with it. Rather, they were pragmatic solutions to specific problems, adapting existing institutions to deal with these.

Box 1.3   Pre-modern policy making: the sixteenth-century Elizabethan Poor Laws

Historical context   Henry VIII's religious reforms involved the dissolution of the monasteries and the loss of their role in providing health and social support for the poor. There was a rapid population growth in the sixteenth century which combined with poor harvests in the 1590s to create serious rural distress and resulted in individuals leaving their home parishes in search of food. In some places these individuals joined others, forming bands of sturdy beggars.

Perceived social problem   Bands of sturdy beggars were seen as a threat to social order.

Process   The issue was raised within the traditional parliamentary system as local problems, i.e. grievances, and 'solved' by a series of Acts of Parliament – 1563, 1572, 1576, 1597 – that were consolidated in the 1601 Act.

Policy outcomes   The 1563 Act confirmed the basic eligibility of the deserving poor for relief in the parish of their legal settlement. The 1572 Act established local poor taxes. The 1576 Act exhorted parishes to establish local workhouses. The 1597 Act created the post of overseer of the poor in each parish. The 1601 Act consolidated the provisions of the previous Acts.

The 1834 New Poor Law was based on a very different approach (see box 1.4). During the 'reform' period of the 1830s, the government appointed an expert Commission to thoroughly examine the causes of, and optimal way of responding to, the problem. This Commission included Bentham's acolyte, Edwin Chadwick, who drew on Bentham's reflections on the Elizabethan Poor Laws – especially his criticism of outdoor relief and his support for a new system of relieving poverty through new model workhouses. The Commission reviewed available evidence and recommended a radical reform of the Poor Law creating an ideal system for managing poverty, using the principle of 'lesser eligibility' to manage the able-bodied poor in new institutions, public workhouses, set within a new administrative structure.

This new system did not 'solve' the problem of poverty; indeed, it created its own problems and critics. For example, romantics such as

> **Box 1.4   Developing modern policy making: the New Poor Law**
>
> *Historical context*   Widespread economic change with shifts in agrarian production, industrial development and population movement to large industrial conurbations; the start of modern cyclical economic development with periods of prosperity alternating with economic downturn and associated unemployment.
>
> *Perceived social problem*   The able-bodied poor were seen as a major social threat, and there were concerns about the rising cost and exploitation of the system of outdoor relief.
>
> *Process*   A committee of experts was appointed to collect evidence and thoroughly review all alternatives and make recommendations. These recommendations were broadly accepted as the basis for the 1834 Poor Law Amendment Act which created a new system of welfare.
>
> *Policy outcomes*   A new system of workhouses based on a clear statement of principles – i.e. lesser eligibility – to ensure that there were strong incentives for thrift and self-reliance and punishment for fecklessness. The aim was to ensure that all relief for the able-bodied poor was provided in workhouses, and that they contributed to their own upkeep by working. The new system involved a substantial expansion of state responsibility and funding.

architect Pugin (Hill 2008) seized upon Bentham's model of the panopticon workhouse as an example of social engineering that deprived individuals of their humanity. By the end of the nineteenth century, such criticisms were generally accepted, but the review and reforms of the system followed the precedent established by the original Commission, i.e. a further expert review making recommendations which formed the basis of government action. In 1905 the reforming Liberal Government appointed a Royal Commission to review the Poor Law. The eighteen commissioners included experts in welfare, and local and national officials. The Commission also included critics who challenged its ideological basis, particularly the Fabian socialists Sidney and Beatrice Webb, who produced and published a minority report that argued the Poor Law needed radical reform, as it was outdated and not appropriate for the contemporary situation (Webb and Webb 1909: ix).

Not only have the overall scope and level of government activity and associated policy making increased substantially over the past 200 years, but so has the rationale for such activity. The prime justification for such policy making is no longer the greater glory of kings and rulers but the greater happiness or increased welfare and well-being of those who are 'ruled'. Contemporary governments are committed to innovation and change in order to create better societies for their citizens, on whose behalf they claim to act and from whom their democratic legitimacy flows (as we will discuss in chapter 7).

1.2 The changing nature of health policy in British government: Changing nature of rationality

Health policy is a major and highly politically sensitive element of government policy. However, in historical terms this has been a relatively recent mid-twentieth-century development. Indeed, as we show in this section, compared to some European countries it was a relatively late development. While this development fits into the 'Enlightenment' programme of enhancing the welfare of citizens, we will argue that dominant health policy concerns have changed. Thus, while all governments have presented their health policies as rational, this rationality has reflected the particular circumstances of different times.

The development of government responsibility for health and health policy

In the United Kingdom, health only emerged as a distinctive area of government policy in the twentieth century, and did so very much as a by-product of other areas of policy. Whereas absolutist states run by 'enlightened despots', such as Prussia, began to take responsibility for the health of their citizens in the eighteenth century (Hennock 1998), until the twentieth century British governments' involvement in health was limited, reflecting a view that the state should as far as possible not intervene in society. There was some involvement but this was a by-product of issues in which the government accepted pressure for intervention, especially relief of the poor and management of the insane.

In the nineteenth century, the government's involvement in health increased with the New Poor Law and Lunacy legislation, through the expansion of the workhouse and lunatic asylums. Both institutions required medical input, to treat sick paupers and to manage the mentally ill. While the numbers were small compared to the general population, the policy implications tended to be broader. When, in 1840, Parliament legislated to make smallpox vaccination free and universal for all children, there were no suitable local authorities to implement the legislation, so the Act required Poor Law Boards of Guardians to appoint qualified medical practitioners to provide free vaccination for *all* infants in all parish unions (Hennock 1998). Such requirements in turn stimulated state involvement in the regulation of the medical profession. When the new workhouses were built in the 1840s, there was no single definitive list of qualified medical practitioners. The utility of having such a list made the Government sympathetic to the medical reform movement (for further discussion, see chapter 9). The Government sponsored the 1854 General Medical Act, effectively creating a single unified medical profession (Parry and Parry 1976).

Although state involvement in medicine grew in the nineteenth century, it did not grow sufficiently for health policy to be recognised as a separate area of policy requiring its own Minister and Ministry. This followed in the early twentieth century when, in 1921, as part of the post-war restructuring of welfare, a Ministry of Health was created. While the establishment of this Ministry reflected increased state involvement in health care, both through the provision of municipal hospitals and through public health departments of local authorities, the remit of the Ministry was broader, taking in the residual poor law system plus an oversight of local government. It was not until 1948, following another World War and further promises of welfare reforms and a welfare state to mobilise support for the war effort, that the Government took on responsibility for the health and health care of the whole population. As part of the formation of the National Health Service in 1948, most non-health responsibilities of the Ministry of Health were transferred to other ministries, and the Minister of Health then focused on the formation and implementation of health policy.

The changing nature of health policy

Since the Government took responsibility for health policy in the 1940s, the prime focus and nature of health policy has changed over time. In the 1940s, with formation of the new health service, health ministers and their civil servants concentrated on running the fledgeling service, especially on ensuring it had enough money. While this has remained an important aspect of policy in Britain, ideological changes, as well as specific events such as disasters, have changed the context of policy making. New areas of health policy have come to the fore.

The formation of the NHS in 1948 is often seen as the basis of modern health care in Britain, but in terms of policy making there was a degree of continuity. The reforms built on and developed the system of decision making which had developed in the early twentieth century, i.e. the medical profession individually and collectively defined the nature of health and health care and controlled the allocation of resources within the new NHS. Central government did act to nationalise the hospitals with a substantial increase in the technical aspects of delivering health care, and related administration of the new service. However, this did not substantially increase the scope of policy making. For much of the 1950s the Ministry of Health remained a civil-service backwater; between Nye Bevan in the 1940s and Enoch Powell in the 1960s, the Minister of Health was effectively a junior minister, and not a full member of the inner elite of ministers, the Cabinet. Ministers and civil servants ran the service in partnership with the medical profession. As Eckstein (1960) documented, British Medical Association (BMA) officials – i.e. officials of the medical professional association – were co-opted into the Ministry of Health and played a lead role in health policy making in this period (we discuss this further in chapters 4 and 6).

There was one important issue which vexed governments in the late 1940s and 1950s, one that could not be dealt with by informal negotiation: money. A key aim of the NHS was to remove the financial burden of illness from the sick person and their family and share it more fairly across society through funding the service from National Insurance and other tax revenues. The formation of the NHS represented a major shift of health-care funding from individuals, local authorities and charities to central government. Webster (1988: 133–83) notes that, following the formation of the NHS on 5 July 1948, there were recurrent crises over the cost of the new service and its funding.

The early architects of the service had accepted that the cost of providing health care would initially rise because of a backlog of ill-health, but argued that once this had been dealt with spending would fall. In February 1948 Bevan requested £198.4 million (gross) for the initial nine months of the service. However, it rapidly became clear that this would not be enough and in a progress report to Cabinet Bevan revised the figures for 1948/9 to £225 million for the nine months, and £330 million for 1949/50. The Treasury had to deal with unplanned additional expenditure creating 'a very big hole through which money has been pouring' (Webster 1988: 151) and was embarrassed by the need to return to Parliament to get approval for further spending. In this context, it is hardly surprising that most visible aspects of health policy making in the first decade of the NHS involved conflicts over money. Bevan as Minister of Health and Stafford Cripps and subsequently Gaitskell as Chancellors clashed over controlling demand and costs through the introduction of charges (this will be discussed further in chapter 3, see box 3.2). Further disagreement existed between Health Ministers and the medical profession over pay which is described in box 1.5.

While the initial tensions and conflicts over the formation of the NHS dissipated in the 1950s, the issues around the cost of health care became a major driver for policy development into the 1960s and beyond (see chapter 3 for a discussion of public expenditure and health care).

As the service settled, so new areas of policy making emerged, reflecting changes in the political environment of policy making and, in particular, renewed interest in investing in and planning public services which were signalled in 1957 by Macmillan, the Conservative Prime Minister, with a speech in which he stated: 'Indeed let us be frank about it – most of our people have never had it so good' (*BBC News* 2008) and signalled the end of post-war austerity. In health the main beneficiaries of new money were the hospitals. Virtually no new hospitals were built in the 1950s and 1960s, so much of the hospital estate was made up of nineteenth-century buildings. Most of the large acute hospitals were located in inner-city areas, most obviously in London, although the populations they served now lived in the suburbs. The precise role and functions of hospitals were not clear. There were many specialist hospitals, some small – such as eye hospitals – located in cities, but most large hospitals in rural areas that had originally been built as lunatic asylums or mental deficiency colonies. Most of these large rural hospitals appeared to be providing long-term social care rather than acute health care and operated under Victorian and Edwardian legislation. They were managed by the Board of Control, a semi-autonomous body that became the Mental Health Division of the Ministry of Health (Webster 1988: 239–40)

**Box 1.5   Policy making in the 1940s: terms and conditions
of general practitioners**

Historical context   Prior to the formation of the NHS, most general
practitioners participated as 'panel doctors' in the 1911 National
Health Insurance scheme which by 1938 provided medical care
for some 20.3 million insured workers. GPs were independent
contractors owning their own premises and receiving a set fee for
each insured worker on their panel. Bevan, the Minister of Health,
aimed to make the scheme universal and to incorporate GPs into
the new NHS as full-time NHS salaried employees working in
NHS premises.

Process   Bevan's predecessors in the wartime Government initiated the key negotiations between the BMA and the Government.
In February 1945 Willink, the Minister of Health, appointed an
academic, Sir Will Spens, to chair an expert committee to advice
on the remuneration of general practitioners. The committee was
invited to estimate the incomes required to protect past standards
and attract suitable recruits to the profession. The committee
included four BMA representatives as well as four independent
experts. A statistician provided expert advice based on a survey of
pre-war earnings of 5,000 GPs. The Report was published in May
1946.

Policy outcome   The committee was concerned by the low pay of
some doctors and the need to attract high-calibre doctors with
prospects of high salaries, so recommended an overall increase in
income with a minimum of £500 per annum for a new entrant,
an average salary of £1,300 for 40- to 50-year-old GPs, and the
prospect of £2,500 for the highest earners. The committee noted
GPs' commitment to the current fee-per-patient system and,
while not recommending any form of payment, based its recommendations on the assumptions that the current system would
continue. The committee effectively gave the BMA the whip-
hand in negotiations, so that not only did GPs get a good salary
settlement, they also retained their status as independent contractors owning their own practices and mainly paid by fees. It also
set the precedent for subsequent independent reviews that made
generous settlements.

when the NHS was set up (see box 5.3 for discussion of reform of the framework of services for patients with mental disorders).

The initial catalyst for the review of hospitals came from an unlikely source, a committee designed to recommend ways of reducing the cost of the new NHS. In November 1952, the Treasury, alarmed about the continuing increase in NHS expenditure decided to appoint an independent inquiry into how the '"rising charge" upon the Exchequer could be avoided' (Webster 1988: 239–40). The Committee was formally established on 1 April 1953 and chaired by Claude Guillebaud, a Cambridge economist. The Committee's report, published on 25 January 1956, did not support the Treasury's case for additional charges and cost control. The Committee argued that there should be more investment in the NHS, especially in hospitals, to increase the efficiency of the service. The Committee noted that the ratio of capital to current expenditure had declined from pre-war years from 19.6 per cent in 1938/9 to 4.1 per cent in 1952/3, while in the USA it was 23.4 per cent in 1951. The Committee recommended that, over a seven-year period, capital expenditure should be increased to £30 million per annum to return to its pre-war level (Webster 1988: 209). Initially the Treasury was not willing to sanction a major increase in spending on hospital building and a major review of hospitals. Increased expenditure on hospitals had to wait until 1960 when a new Minister, Enoch Powell was able to negotiate a major programme of investment with the Treasury (see Allen 1979). Box 1.6 highlights the rational elements of the plan (but note that in box 3.4 we offer an alternative interpretation of this plan).

The Hospital Plan focused on the needs of acute patients, and less attention was paid to the situation of those individuals who required long-term care, until in the late 1960s, when a series of claims about scandalous conditions in long-term hospitals resulted in investigations and prompted a series of policy initiatives to improve such care (in chapter 5 we discuss the role of disasters in the formation of health policy).

In the late 1960s there were also major changes in the machinery of government (we discuss these further in chapter 2) which created the political will and capacity to expand the scope of policy making. In 1968 the Labour Government created a 'superministry', the Department of Health and Social Security, led by a minister with oversight for all government social policy. Richard Crossman, an experienced 'heavy-weight' Labour politician was the first Secretary of State for Social Services, and when Labour were defeated in 1970, he was replaced by Sir Keith Joseph, one of the key architects of the

---

Box 1.6   Policy making in the 1960s: the rational planning of modern hospitals

Historical context   A period of economic growth coincided with a Conservative Government led by Harold Macmillan committed to modernisation of the public and private sectors through systematic planning. There was awareness of underinvestment in hospitals.

Process   A combination of expert evidence and opinion with political negotiation was involved. Evidence for the more efficient use of hospital beds came from visits to the USA plus studies in Oxford in 1957 and Barrow in 1960, indicating that an efficient service could be provided with 2 to 2.5 beds per 1,000 population – a reduction from wartime estimates of 4.6 to 6 beds per 1,000. Expert opinion came from the BMA which published several reports recommending ten-year investment of £750 million. Ministry of Health negotiations with the Treasury were aided by appointments of Enoch Powell as Minister of Health and Bruce Fraser as Permanent Secretary in the Ministry of Health. Both had had experience of working in the Treasury.

Policy outcome   The Hospital Plan was published on 23 January 1962. Powell and Fraser had secured £500 million of investment for hospitals over ten years to build 90 new hospitals and re-model another 134. The Plan introduced the concept of the district general hospital (DGH) which was to be more efficient and use fewer beds than the specialist hospitals it replaced. DGHs were to have between 600 and 800 beds, contain a comprehensive range of acute specialist hospital services, including psychiatric and geri-atric services as well as Consultant-led maternity units, and serve between 100,000 and 150,000 people.

New Right ideology and 1980s Thatcherism. In 1971 the Department was reorganised, creating specialist teams of professionals and civil servants who focused on the policy relating to specific service users or 'client groups' (we discuss these further in chapter 2, and we discuss the disasters which prompted policy developments for some of these client groups in chapter 5). Following the review of policy for people with learning disabilities (see box 1.7) – *Better Services for the Mentally Handicapped* (Department of Health and Social Security 1971) – the Department of Health and Social Security produced a series of policy

---

Box 1.7   Policy making in the 1970s: improving services for people with learning disabilities

Historical context   In the 1960s there was investment in new 'mental handicap' hospitals and there were developments of new local authority services such as residential homes and adult training centres. Civil servants were aware that some hospitals did not provide adequate standards of care but this evidence was not passed on to Ministers.

Process   Following allegations of abuses at Ely Hospital, Cardiff, the Minister of Health commissioned an independent inquiry. The Inquiry not only substantiated the allegations but drew attention to the lack of clear policy guidance from central government. The incoming Secretary of State, Richard Crossman, accepted responsibility for policy failure and commissioned an independent group to review policy for people with learning disabilities.

Policy outcome   The recommendations of the review group were accepted by Crossman's successor, Sir Keith Joseph, and formed the basis of a major policy statement, *Better Services for the Mentally Handicapped* (Department of Health and Social Security 1971). The policy involved a major reconfiguration of services with the closure of all long-stay hospitals and the development of community services.

---

statements outlining policies for specific client groups, such as *Better Services for the Mentally Ill* (Department of Health and Social Security 1975) and *A Happier Old Age* (Department of Health and Social Security and the Welsh Office 1978).

The early development of health policy was focused very much on service delivery, with initial concerns about the cost of the service leading on to concerns about the quality of and investment in acute services and then services for deprived service users. The search for efficiency and value for money remained a policy concern and stimulated repeated restructuring of the NHS. However, as the NHS became well established by the 1970s, so ministers' aspirations moved beyond just running the service efficiently towards using health policy as a mechanism of social reform and as a way of creating a better, healthier and fairer society. Implicit in this shift was an increased emphasis on public health and a broader commitment to the health of the nation.

The shift in aspirations from just providing health care to enhancing the health of all citizens was incremental, starting in 1974, when the Department of Health and Social Security accepted that the reorganised NHS should seek to prevent as well as treat disease, and culminating in 1992, when the Government published the first of the *Health of the Nation* White Papers.

In the 1950s, epidemiologists such as Sir Richard Doll drew attention to the link between smoking and lung cancer, and public health specialists such as Thomas McKeown (1979) identified the major role which environmental factors had played in improvements in health in the nineteenth and twentieth centuries. However, the Government's most senior medical adviser, the Chief Medical Officer (CMO), in a memorandum written in 1955 to the Guillebaud Committee, stated that it was unlikely that research into preventative approaches would make any major improvement in the country's health and felt there were 'no new fields for preventative action' (Webster 1988: 377).

The restructuring of the NHS in 1974 stimulated preventative medicine, moving public health from the backwater of local government to the centre of local decision making (see Haywood and Alaszewski 1980). Before the reorganisation, local authorities had health departments run by Medical Officers of Health which provided some preventative services, but public health was neglected in both the medical profession and the NHS. The reorganisation of the NHS created strategic Area Health Authorities and operational District Management Teams. Public-health doctors became key players as Area Medical Officers and District Community Physicians. While most of their time and energy was devoted to managing the new system, they did also create and manage new preventative services, stimulating the development of a new type of activity with its own specialist staff and expertise, health promotion.

The development of public health and health promotion in the NHS was matched by increasing government awareness of their importance. The development of client-group policy-making teams increased awareness amongst policy makers of the health implications of lifestyle choices such as overeating or consuming legal and illegal drugs. Such problems could only be addressed by persuading individuals to change their behaviour, thus the first review of policy on alcohol was called *Drinking Sensibly* (Department of Health and Social Security 1981). Government interest in behaviour and prevention was further stimulated by the emergence of new infectious diseases, especially HIV/AIDS in the early 1980s (see chapter 9). By 1985 it was clear that HIV was a sexually transmitted disease and it

---

**Box 1.8   Policy making in the 1990s: focusing on the
health of the nation**

Historical context   Following the resignation of the Conservative
Prime Minister Margaret Thatcher in 1990, her successor John
Major and an increasingly unpopular Conservative Government
sought ways of increasing popularity and persuading the public
that they were committed to the NHS.

Process   Health ministers asked their chief medical adviser, the
Chief Medical Officer, to review evidence on national and international developments in health promotion, and the report of
his expert working group formed the basis of a Green Paper
(Department of Health 1991a) that identified sixteen potential areas
for action. Following consultation, the Secretary of State published
a White Paper, *Health of the Nation* (Department of Health 1992).

Policy outcome   The White Paper established targets for measurable health gains, creating a strategy for the NHS and for other
public services. The aim was to reduce ill-health in five key areas:
coronary heart disease and stroke, cancer, mental illness, HIV/
AIDS and sexual health, and accidents. Each area had a statement of main objectives and there were twenty-seven targets for
improvement across the five areas. In 1997 the incoming Labour
Government commissioned an academic review of the strategy
(Department of Health 1998a), which concluded that it had not
been fully successful, and its subsequent policy statements (e.g.
Saving Lives – Department of Health 1999a) refined the strategy,
adding a focus on social justice.

---

was anticipated that the disease would spread rapidly from high-risk
groups to the rest of the population. The Secretary of State for Social
Services, Sir Norman Fowler, persuaded his Cabinet colleagues that
the best way of managing the new disease was through a high-profile
health promotion campaign to make the population aware of the risk
and persuade them to adopt safer sexual practices.

   As local and central government interest in public health and health
promotion developed piecemeal through the 1980s, there was no
overall statement on the role and purpose of such activities. In the
1990s, the Secretary of State, Virginia Bottomley rectified this by
issuing a new White Paper (Department of Health 1992; see box 1.8).

Improving the overall health of the population through the provision of health care and public information has become one of the 'big ideas' and major objectives of health policy makers. It is very much in the utilitarian tradition of maximising the benefits gained from government action by increasing happiness – or, in this case, health. It is possible to identify another related policy objective that focuses more explicitly on the NHS: the minimisation of the harm caused by the health service and its staff.

Since the provision of health care is intrinsically risky – for example, acute hospitals are trying to treat people who are often seriously ill, and mental health services treat people who may be dangerous to themselves and others – the outcomes may be harm to the patient or others. Sometimes this harm is the result of error or negligence. In the first phase of the NHS, there was little official interest in such preventable harm. For example, Webster (1988), in his official history of the NHS, does not discuss negligence or error. The courts were unsympathetic to negligence claims against the NHS and the fledgeling service was to some degree protected from health and safety prosecutions by Crown immunity (in chapter 5 we discuss the ways in which the early NHS was insulated from the consequences of medical errors).

By the 1990s there was increased concern and evidence that treatment by the NHS caused some patients harm. In 2001 the results of a retrospective review of records indicated that 11.7 per cent of the patients treated in the NHS experienced preventable harm (see Vincent, Neale and Woloshynowych 2001). Furthermore, individuals seemed more willing to sue and courts more willing to award damages for negligence. Fenn and his colleagues explored the changing pattern of negligence by analysing the database of medical negligence claims of Oxfordshire Health Authority. They identified an increasing propensity to claim (a rise from 0.46 to 0.86 closed claims per 1,000 finished Consultant episodes between 1990 and 1998) and rising costs (from £52.3 million in 1990/1 to £84 million in 1998). They estimated that the overall NHS liability for negligence claims was in the order of £1.8 billion (Fenn, Hermans and Dingwall 1994; Fenn et al. 2000). In 2001, the Department of Health identified four areas in which there is a regular pattern of errors, and targeted these for improvement: maladministered spinal injections; obstetrics and gynaecology; errors in the use of prescribed drugs; and suicides by hanging from non-collapsible rails on wards (Department of Health 2001a: 45).

Box 1.9   Policy making in the 2000s: quality, risk and clinical governance

Hisorical context   In 1997 a new Labour Government was elected, with a substantial majority and a 'New Labour' agenda. The Chancellor of the Exchequer was committed to maintaining the spending plans of the outgoing Conservative Government which ruled out an immediate large increase in public spending. Frank Dobson, a politician reaching the end of his career, was a surprise appointment as Secretary of State. He was considered a stop-gap to enable more junior colleagues such as Alan Milburn (Minister of Health) to acquire more experience. The incoming ministers needed to achieve a difficult balance: to make major innovations without a substantial increase in spending.

Process   Milburn conducted a review of existing policies for the NHS, especially the internal market. With a bit of renaming and restructuring, these policies were retained. The review focused on safety and decision making in the NHS.

Policy outcome   The White Paper, *The New NHS: Modern, Dependable* (Department of Health 1997), put in place a framework which included clinical governance, changes in professional regulation, national service frameworks and the National Institute for Clinical Excellence, and the Commission for Health Improvement to improve the quality of decision making in the NHS and to ensure patient safety.

There were also a series of well-documented health disasters, including unacceptable paediatric heart surgery failure rates at Bristol Royal Infirmary, and the failure to identify the harmful activities of the general practitioner Harold Shipman (we discuss these in more detail in chapter 5). As part of the post-1997 'modernisation' strategy, the Labour Government pledged to develop a more effective system of risk management. The Government clearly articulated a commitment to an NHS that protected its patients and had systems to 'minimise the risk to . . . patients and improve the quality and safety of patient care' (Department of Health 2000a: 90). The key elements of the modernisation strategy are discussed in box 1.9.

Comment

Since the nineteenth century, UK government has expanded in both scope and size, and since 1945 has claimed to provide care and protection for all its citizens through a welfare state. While the British political system has retained traditional elements, the rationale for government action is derived from eighteenth- and nineteenth-century Enlightenment thinkers. Policy makers use knowledge to create a better future. Through continual reform and improvement, they try to create changes that will increase collective benefit or enhance the greatest happiness of the greatest number of citizens.

KEY POINTS

- Policy making is a key part of government activity and is a process of identifying the aims of government and the best way of achieving them.
- As government activities have changed and expanded, so have the nature of, and rationale for, policy making.
- In the premodern period, the scope of government activity was relatively limited and innovations in policy came primarily from pressure to redress individual or collective grievances. Thus, policy making mainly took the form of law making and was justified as the restatement of traditional customs and practices, rather than the reform of social relations and institutions.
- Since the eighteenth century, Enlightenment thinking has provided the rationale for government action. Policy making is seen and justified in terms of modernisation, i.e. reform and improvement, and as a way of creating changes in relations and institutions that will increase collective benefit or enhance the greatest happiness of the greatest number.
- Modern policy making involves defining worthwhile ends for government action, i.e. appraising and agreeing which visions of the future are worth pursuing, as well as evaluating the best ways of achieving such visions.
- Utilitarianism, with its emphasis on instrumental rationality and efficiency and fairness, both legitimates and shapes modern policy making. By providing knowledge about the benefits of different approaches, utilitarianism ensures that the most effective use is made of the resources which society provides for public services. The use of independent 'objective' experts means that irrelevant

factors, such as prejudice against certain individuals or groups within society, can be filtered out and resources allocated to meet the needs which individuals have.

- In the UK, health policy making was formally recognised in 1921 with the formation of a Ministry of Health, but it was only in the 1940s, with the formation of the NHS, that health became the prime focus of the Ministry.
- Since the formation of the NHS, ministers and their advisers have taken on responsibility for providing health care for the UK populations. While this policy making has always been rational, as circumstances have changed, so has the nature of this rationality:

1948–68 – Running an efficient health service – controlling the costs of the service and making investments to enhance its quality.

1968–90 – Responding to changing demand and health problems – dealing with disasters such as scandals in hospitals, and new diseases such as HIV/AIDS.

Post-1990 – Improving the health of citizens and protecting them from harm – the concern with the efficient and effective operation of the NHS broadened to focus on the collective benefits of government policy, especially improving the health of the nation, saving lives and creating a safe NHS.

PART 1
Rationality in Policy Making

2

Managing knowledge and expertise: attempting to create rational health policy

AIMS

To examine the importance of knowledge in rational policy making and to consider ways of dealing with the challenges for governments in accessing and using appropriate knowledge, and how they have responded to such challenges.

OBJECTIVES

- To consider the importance of the effective use of scientific knowledge and expertise in rational health policy making
- To identify the challenges in the UK, especially the knowledge gap that results from appointment of key policy makers – ministers – who do not have expertise in the domain of health
- To consider the ways in which policy issues are logically grouped together and the relative stability of those grouped around health
- To examine the impact which the search for better knowledge and expertise has had on the machinery of health policy making in the UK.

In chapter 1 we noted the ways in which contemporary governments seek to justify their actions and policies in terms of the rationality of their policies and the benefits which these policies create for citizens. In this chapter we develop this analysis by examining the importance of scientific knowledge in rational policy making and the knowledge deficit that results from the appointment in the UK of ministers who have political expertise but not necessarily any specialist knowledge of the policy area they are responsible for. We consider the ways this problem is overcome through the use of advisers, and the on-going search for improvements in access to expertise and knowledge.

2.1 Rationality in policy making: using appropriate knowledge

In the Enlightenment programme the rationality of government action is defined in terms of instrumentality, i.e. as the best means of achieving specified ends. Such instrumental rationality is grounded in scientific knowledge of the best ends or outcome and the most effective way of achieving the desired outcome. The American sociologist Talcott Parsons argued that policy is rational: 'in so far as it pursues ends possible within the conditions of the situation, and by the means which, among those available to [the policy maker], are intrinsically best adapted to the ends for reasons understandable and verifiable by positive empirical science' (Parsons 1949: 58).

Simon identified the processes underlying rational policy making in the following way:

> the work that steers the course of society and its economic and governmental organisations – is largely work of making decisions and solving problems. It is work of *choosing issues that require attention, setting goals, finding or designing suitable courses of action, and evaluating and choosing among alternative actions.* The first three of these activities – fixing agendas, setting goals, and designing actions – are usually called *problem solving*; the last, evaluating and choosing, is usually called *decision making*. Nothing is more important for the well-being of society than that this work be performed effectively, that we address successfully the many problems requiring attention at the national level (the budget and trade deficits, AIDS, national security, the mitigation of earthquake damage). (Simon 1986: 1, italics added)

Simon argued that it is possible to consider the best way of approaching such problems and to identify systems that will maximise benefit, i.e. specify 'the conditions of perfect utility-maximizing rationality in a world of certainty' (1986: 1). His caveat that policy making can only be rational in a world of certainty acknowledges that in reality there is uncertainty, i.e. an absence of full knowledge, and that policy makers need to improve policy making by improving their access to knowledge.

Simon argued that rationality involves a sequence of activity starting with the identification of a policy problem, and moving through

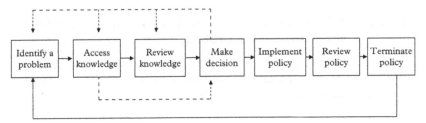

Figure 2.1 A diagrammatic representation of a rational policy-making
system Adapted from Jenkins 1978:17

the identification and evaluation of alternative ways of dealing with
the problem to decision making and policy implementation. Jenkins
(1978) represented rational policy making as a series of activities
linked by feedback loops. The main loop leads from the termination
of one policy to the start of the next as shown in figure 2.1.

While both Simon and Jenkins indicate that rational policy making
starts with either choosing issues or identifying a problem, there is
actually little discussion of how such issues or problems are identified. The implication in rational planning is that ends are defined in
the same way as the evaluation of means, i.e. through the accumulation of knowledge. However, as we will show in chapter 6 when
we focus more closely on the ways in which issues, problems or the
desired ends of policy making are determined, it becomes clear that
knowledge is neither sufficient nor necessary.

In the Enlightenment programme, policy is only rational if there
is full or at least adequate knowledge about the nature of social
problems, the possible responses to such problems and the probable outcomes of these responses. Policy makers need to draw on
the knowledge created by scientific investigation, but where this is
inadequate they need to create additional knowledge, for example
by funding the scientific investigation of practical problems. As we
will discuss in chapters 5 and 9, policy makers are under pressure to
respond quickly to new problems and often do not consider they have
the time to commission and respond to new knowledge (Toynbee
2010). Creating new knowledge means resisting the Enlightenment
imperative to take action. For example, in the case of HIV/AIDS
in the early 1980s and vCJD in the early 1990s policy makers were
criticised for inaction, even though they had commissioned scientific
research that identified the nature of the new diseases (see box 2.1 for
HIV/AIDS, and, for vCJD, box 5.1).

This emphasis on acquiring and using appropriate knowledge
and expertise reflects a concern to use available resources in the

---

Box 2.1   HIV/AIDS: using scientific knowledge to establish the nature of the problem

Historical context   In the early 1980s a new disease was identified, initially on the West Coast of the USA and subsequently in major cities in Europe. It appeared to be associated mainly with men who have sex with other men and there was considerable media coverage with a strong moralising dimension.

Process   The Conservative Government provided additional monies for the Medical Research Council to fund scientific investigation into the nature and causes of the new disease.

Outcome   By 1985 the disease was identified as Acquired Immune Deficiency Syndrome (AIDS) and the consensus of scientific opinion was that it was caused by the Human Immunodeficiency Virus (HIV) which spread through bodily fluids especially blood, via sexual activity, sharing of intravenous injection equipment and contaminated Factor VIII clotting agent. Such knowledge underpinned the development of various preventative measures.

---

most effective and rational manner and also to minimise irrational and arbitrary influences. The Department for the Environment, Food and Rural Affairs (DEFRA) has advocated an evidence-based policy-making system that counteracts 'short-term political pressures' through the use of evidence.

> The key benefit of evidence-based policy making is better policy. The recent increase in interest in evidence-based policy making comes in response to a perception that Government needs to improve the quality of decision-making . . . Many critics argued in the past that policy decisions were too often driven by inertia or by short-term political pressures. There are many different definitions of the term 'evidence based policy making' but we use it here to refer to an *approach* to policy development and implementation which uses rigorous techniques to develop and maintain a robust evidence base from which to develop policy options. (DEFRA n.d.)

The main elements of this system are presented in figures 2.2 and 2.3.

In the rational model, policy makers should be objective experts who apply reason and knowledge to identify society's problems

There are policy options that...

Use good information...   ...and use it well...

Use poor information...   ...and use it poorly...

Figure 2.2   DEFRA assessment of the use of information in policy
Source: DEFRA

Longer-term policy and strategy development

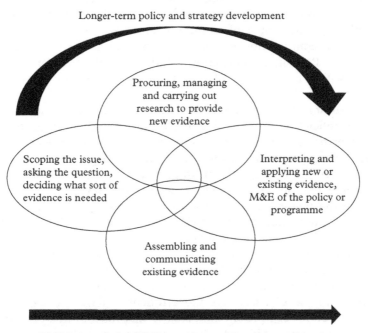

Procuring, managing
and carrying out
research to provide
new evidence

Scoping the issue,
asking the question,
deciding what sort of
evidence is needed

Interpreting and
applying new or
existing evidence,
M&E of the policy or
programme

Assembling and
communicating
existing evidence

Evidence needed rapidly to answer pressing policy questions

Figure 2.3   The use of evidence in policy making
Source: DEFRA

and make decisions that create maximum social benefit. Thus, for advocates of rational policy making, the key to good policy making is appropriate knowledge that is effectively analysed. The Haldane Inquiry in 1918 into the operation of government emphasised the importance of 'investigation and thought as a preliminary to action' (Hennessy 1990: 297). However, as we will show in the next section, there is a major problem in policy making in the UK as the key group of policy makers, government ministers, are not appointed because of their expertise – or even interest – in a particular policy area.

2.2 A knowledge deficit: ministers and their policy expertise

Ministers are key policy makers and the public face of policy. They are responsible for publicly stating and explaining policy decisions. As we discuss in chapter 9, this involves explaining such policies to and through the media. Since the United Kingdom is a democracy, the public is represented by Members of Parliament, and therefore ministers have to present and explain their policies to Parliament. Hence the convention in the United Kingdom that ministers must be Members of the House of Commons or Lords: 'The basic requirement of accountability is that ministers explain their actions and policies to Parliament, and inform Parliament of events or developments within their sphere of responsibility' (Powell and Gay 2004: 7).

Since ministers are responsible for the formation and implementation of policies within specified areas, they should apologise for and rectify errors if these result from their policies. When the errors and their consequences are serious, they should resign. However, there is considerable dispute about what exactly constitutes an 'error', especially one so serious that it necessitates resignation. Indeed, despite the major health disasters which we examine in chapter 5, such as murders committed by Harold Shipman and Beverley Allitt, there have been lots of apologies but very few resignations. Of the 125 ministerial resignations in the twentieth century, only one was in the area of health: Edwina Currie (see Powell and Gay 2004: 35–7). In a radio programme in December 1988, Currie, a junior health minister in the Conservative Government, referred to widespread concerns about egg production, stating that most of this production was contaminated with salmonella, resulting in a slump in sales of eggs. She was forced to resign – probably to ensure government relations with egg producers could be restored (Powell and Gay 2004: 27).

The importance of ministers as the public face of policy creates a major paradox. Ministers, particularly in the UK government system, are usually successful politicians but they have little experience of policy making and limited knowledge of the substantive area for which they become responsible. As Dror noted: 'The nature of political competition in democracies emphasises criteria that have little correlation with the qualities needed for some of the main tasks of rulers, especially policy-making' (1987: 191). Prime Ministers, who appoint ministers in the UK, have a small pool of people to select from. In 2008 the Government was made up 118 ministers, of whom 25 were in the House of Lords and 93 in the House of Commons (Cabinet Office 2008). Most of the senior ministers (members of the Cabinet) were in the Commons (21 out of 23). Thus, when choosing senior ministers and most junior ministers, the Prime Minister is restricted to Members of Parliament who accept the government whip, i.e. between 325 and 425 Members of Parliament who belong to the party – or in the case of the 2010 election, coalition of parties – that won the preceding general election. However, the Prime Minister can extend his options by making appointments to the House of Lords. In 2007, when he became Prime Minister, Gordon Brown appointed non-party peers to his government of 'all talents' (Brown and Morris 2007), including Professor the Lord Darzi of Denham as a junior health minister, who is profiled in box 2.2.

The Prime Minister needs to ensure that his or her government team can effectively present and defend government policies and that it includes all key politicians within the party. Hence it is unlikely that many ministers, when appointed, will have particular knowledge of the policy area for which they are responsible. In many European countries, it is common practice for the minister responsible for health policy to have relevant expertise, i.e. be a doctor. In the United Kingdom none of the Secretaries of State since 1968 have been medically qualified. Virginia Bottomley, Secretary of State for Health from 1992 to 1995, however, did have professional training as a social worker and expertise in policy issues as a social scientist and former researcher for Child Poverty Action Group. There have been Ministers of State with medical qualifications, the most famous being Dr David Owen from 1974 to 1976.

The lack of both interest and expertise was evident in the case of Sir Norman Fowler. He came from a private-sector background and made it clear that he was interested in policy making relating to this sector. When the Conservatives were elected in 1979, the Prime Minister, Margaret Thatcher, acknowledged this interest and gave him responsibility for Transport. In 1981 when she culled the 'wets' in her Cabinet she unexpectedly offered Fowler responsibility for health and social services. He publicly stated that he knew nothing about social policy but accepted the post. Despite his limited interest and expertise, he retained the post of Secretary of State for Social Services until after the 1987 election when he was offered the post of Secretary of State for Employment.

Health ministers generally have very limited specialist knowledge of health. In 2008 there were six health ministers in England

(Department of Health 2008a). In box 2.2 we provide profiles for two of these ministers: Alan Johnson, with a typical political career and limited health background, and Lord Darzi who had an atypical background. Of the six ministers in 2008, only two of the junior ministers, Lord Darzi and Ann Keen, had experience of working in the NHS, but both these junior ministers were appointed for their commitment to the New Labour programme of health reforms.

The Coalition Government elected in 2010 showed some differences from the normal pattern of ministerial appointments. There were only five health ministers in England, and only one junior minister had experience of working in the NHS. Ann Milton had relatively little experience of parliamentary politics – she was first elected to Parliament in 2005, but she was a nurse who had twenty-five years' experience of working in the NHS (Department of Health 2010a). Since the Government was a coalition of the Conservative and Liberal Democrat parties, the ministerial team was made up of four Conservatives and a Liberal Democrat, Paul Burstow, Minister of State for Care Services (Department of Health 2010b). Although the ministerial team had little experience of working in health or social care or of making health policy, they did have substantial experience of criticising the health policy of the preceding Labour Government as opposition spokespeople. For example, Andrew Lansley, who became Secretary of State for Health in May 2010, had been Conservative spokesman on health since 2003 (Department of Health 2010c). This meant that when he was appointed Andrew Lansley had clear ideas on how he wanted to reform the NHS, but regrettably he and his team lacked ministerial experience, which meant that they did not have equivalent skills in selling their reforms. As a result, in April 2011, the Prime Minister, David Cameron, announced an unprecedented two-month pause in the legislative process for further consultation (National Health Executive 2011), which we discuss further in the final section of chapter 4. The pressure for this pause partly came from the Liberal Democrat Party which seemed to be taking much of the blame for the unpopularity of Coalition policies. As a result of the pause its leader, the Deputy Prime Minister Nick Clegg, was able to promise '"substantive change" to the reforms to address concerns, including on the governance of GP consortia, the role of the private sector in the NHS, and the detail on accountability and transparency' (National Health Executive 2011).

Box 2.2   Experience and responsibilities of two Health Ministers in England in 2008 (source: Department of Health 2008a)

Alan Johnson: Secretary of State for Health (2007–2009)

Responsibilities   NHS and social care delivery and system reforms; finance and resources; strategic communications.

Reasons for appointment   Alan Johnson was a senior Labour Party politician with strong links to the Labour movement and legitimacy as former Trade Union leader. He was a potential rival to the Prime Minister, Gordon Brown, so giving him a senior Cabinet post ensured that an important part of the Labour party was represented in Cabinet with a possible rival co-opted and a potential threat minimised.

Biography   Alan Johnson was born in 1950 and was educated at Sloane Grammar School, Chelsea. He became a postman in 1968. He was active in the trade union movement, initially in the Communication Workers Union (CWU), where he held a number of posts from 1976. He was elected to the National Executive Council in 1981, became General Secretary in 1992 and Joint General Secretary of the Communication Workers Union from 1995 to 1997. He was a Member of the General Council, TUC, from 1994 to 1995.

He became an MP for Hull East in 1997. As a backbencher he joined the Trade and Industry Select Committee. His involvement in government started in 1997 when he took on the role of Parliamentary Private Secretary for Dawn Primarolo, who was Financial Secretary in the Treasury. His ministerial career started with posts in Trade and Industry (1999–2003) and Education and Skills (2003–4). He was in the Cabinet from 2004 to 2010 as Secretary of State for Work and Pensions (2004–5), Secretary of State for Trade and Industry (2005–6) and Secretary of State for Education and Skills (2006–7), before in June 2007 being appointed Secretary of State for Health. In June 2009 he was appointed Home Secretary when Jacqui Smith unexpectedly resigned, and when the Labour Government was defeated in 2010 he became shadow Chancellor for a short period.

Professor the Lord Darzi of Denham: Parliamentary Under Secretary of State (2007–2009)

Responsibilities NHS next-stage review; quality and innovation; the National Institute for Health and Clinical Excellence (NICE).

Reasons for appointment Co-opting Lord Darzi, a distinguished medical practitioner, into the government was a way of providing professional endorsement for the NHS reform programme, but the experiment was not a whole-hearted success as Lord Darzi lasted only two years.

Biography Ara Warkes Darzi, Baron Darzi of Denham, was born in 1960 in Iraq in a family with a Christian Armenian background. He moved to Ireland in 1977 and studied medicine at the undergraduate facility of the Royal College of Surgeons in Ireland and obtained a Doctor of Medicine degree from Trinity College, Dublin. He moved to the UK to practise medicine and was naturalised in 2002. He is a Consultant surgeon at St Mary's Hospital in the Imperial College Healthcare NHS Trust and the Royal Marsden NHS Foundation Trust and specialises in keyhole surgery. The work of his team has been recognised with international awards and Darzi's personal contribution to surgery and medicine was recognised in 2002 with a knighthood. He was given a peerage in 2007 and appointed by Gordon Brown on 29 June 2007 to his government of 'all talents'. He undertook various reviews for the NHS, including a review of the health-care needs of Londoners (Darzi 2007) and reviews of the NHS (2008a and 2008b). He did not last the full term and resigned his post on 14 July 2009.

2.3 Rationally grouping policy issues: ministers and their ministries

Policy makers do not focus on a single issue but have to deal with a multiplicity of complex issues. Given the complexity and range of potential policy issues and the relatively small number of ministers, policy making can only be rational if ministers are responsible for issues that can be logically grouped together and share common characteristics. As we noted in chapter 1, since the early twentieth century, health has formed a distinctive area of government policy although the precise issues included and boundaries of health policy have changed over time. A senior minister, the Secretary of State for Health, is responsible for health policy in England. The devolution of policy making to ministers in Scotland, Wales and Northern Ireland means that there are separate health ministers, each of whom is accountable to their Parliament or Assembly.

Since England is the largest country within the UK, its ministerial team has traditionally played a leading role in UK health policy making. As a result, health policy across the UK tends to be similar but there are important differences in details. Prescription charges have since the early stages been contentious in the NHS (as we show in box 3.2) and the health ministers in the different parts of the UK have adopted different policies. In Wales, prescription charges for medicines were abolished on 1 April 2007 (National Health Service Wales n.d.). In Scotland, the prescription charge was reduced from £6.85 to £5.00 on 1 April 2008 and abolished on 1 April 2011, while in Northern Ireland it was frozen at £6.85 and then abolished in 2010. In England, on 1 April 2008, the prescription charge was raised from £6.85 to £7.10, rising to £7.40 on 1 April 2011.

The changing definition and boundaries of health

As we noted in chapter 1, having a minister with named responsibility for health is a relatively recent development in the evolution of government in the UK. It seems relatively self-evident that there should be at least one minister with responsibility for health. However, this responsibility has at times been combined with responsibilities for other major areas of policy making. From 1968 (when Richard Crossman took over responsibility for the new super ministry, the Department of Health and Social Security) until 1987 when the Prime Minister, Margaret Thatcher, decided it was too much for one person, the Secretary of State for Social Services was responsible for health and associated policy making as well as social security policy making. In Scotland, the Cabinet Secretary for Health and Welfare was in 2008 the Deputy First Minister and, in addition to the usual elements of health policy, her responsibilities included sport, anti-poverty measures, housing and regeneration (The Scottish Government 2008).

Thus the boundaries of policy-making responsibilities can shift, and those of 'health policy' have both expanded and contracted in England (see box 2.3 for the changing responsibility for policy making in relation to the social care of children).

The basic map of policy-making responsibilities which developed through the nineteenth and twentieth centuries was grounded in the rational principle that a minister or group of ministers should be responsible for a major government task or function – whether this was economic policy (the Chancellor of the Exchequer), law and order (the Home Secretary) or the health of the nation (the respective health ministers in England, Scotland, Wales and Northern Ireland). However, as Brown and Steel (1979) pointed out this principle can be interpreted in different ways.

As we note in box 2.3, decisions about and making policy for the social care needs of looked-after children does not fit easily with thinking about ways of managing adult offenders, as it was supposed to do in the 1960s, but it can equally well be considered together with the social care needs of families – as it was from 1971 until 2008 – or with the educational needs of all children, as it was after 2008. The lack of a definitive map of government tasks, and clear boundaries between categories of tasks, means that there is in practice a continual realignment of policy areas. Brown and Steel (1979) reviewed the alignment of policy areas in the late 1960s and 1970s and suggested that, while the main outline of the map of policy areas had remained relatively constant, there had been substantial changes both in the detailed grouping of issues and also in the names given to the ministers and departments responsible for these areas, which ensured that sign writers were kept busy. For example, following the formation of the Coalition Government in May 2010, one of the first decisions of the Conservative/Liberal Coalition was to change the name of the Department of Children, Schools and Families to the Department of Education to mark a clear break with Ed Ball's period as Secretary of State. This change reflected a shift in the symbolism of policy making from the expansive and modern tone of Ed Ball's department with its child-friendly rainbow logo to a more formal and traditional approach (Shepherd 2010).

In some ways the grouping of issues in health policy is logical and therefore rational. Since the formation of the NHS in 1948 there have been a group of health ministers who have dealt with issues relating to health and health care. However, there are also more arbitrary and therefore less rational elements. The devolution of government in the United Kingdom has resulted in a fragmentation of the NHS and of health policy making into four countries with four separate sets of ministers and departments. While England is largest

---

Box 2.3   Changing responsibility for the social care of children

The 1960s: outside the health portfolio   For historical reasons, the Home Office was responsible for the care of children who were 'looked after' because they did not have parents or their parents had not provided adequate care. The Children's Service of the Home Office regulated the activities of children's departments within local authorities. Social workers played a lead role in developing and delivering these services.

The 1970s: into the health portfolio   In 1968, the Seebohm Committee recommended the formation in England of personal social services departments bringing together social care services, including those for children. The Home Secretary (James Callaghan) and Secretary of State for Social Services (Richard Crossman) agreed that the Department of Health and Social Security should be responsible for policy making when the new local authority social services department started work in 1971.

The 2000s: transfer to education   In 2008 in the continued search for policies to prevent child abuse, the Government issued further guidance that each local authority should create a Trust based on a partnership of all local services, which would produce local childcare plans with targets, and that in due course the Government would give such Trusts a separate legal identity as statutory bodies (DCSF 2008). Given the development of a single partnership to deliver children's services in localities, it followed that a single ministry should provide oversight and policy development. Given the centrality of local authorities and schools, it was agreed that Ed Balls the Secretary of State for Children, Schools and Families and a close colleague of the Prime Minister, should take on this responsibility.

---

and tends to take the lead, there are differences in policies and levels of funding between the four countries. Furthermore, the boundaries of health policies have shifted. In the early 1970s health expanded to include social care, reflecting perceptions that health and social care were and should be interdependent and aspirations that the emergence of social work would facilitate the development of social services modelled on the NHS, i.e. to generate and use knowledge to identify and manage social problems such as child abuse. The 2008 realignment of the boundaries between health and education policy in which the responsibility for policy relating to children needing social care moved from 'health' to 'education' marked the end of these aspirations.

2.4 Accessing knowledge: political advisers and civil servants

Given their relative lack of specific knowledge of the issues in the areas for which they are responsible, especially when they are newly appointed, ministers need ways of accessing expertise and knowledge. As the Haldane Committee noted in 1918, a minister must have 'an organization sufficient to provide him with a general survey of existing knowledge on any subject within his sphere' (quoted in Brown and Steele 1979: 250). Such a survey can come from the special advisers that ministers bring with them into government and from the expertise of the civil servants in their department.

Special advisers

There has been a major expansion of special advisers since the 1960s. All ministers have made use of expert aides but Prime Ministers have made particular use of them as this post is not supported by a ministry. The 1997 Labour Government used sixty-five advisers. Blair, the Prime Minister from 1997 to 2007, effectively set up a policy unit to give him advice on policy issues being considered by ministers and their departments. He had weekly meetings with policy advisers including Alistair Campbell (press) and Jonathan Powell (Chief of Staff) and he also had bright young civil servants seconded from their departments to provide him with more detailed advice.

Special advisers provide a trusted and independent source of advice and are particularly important when Ministers want to make major innovations that are not seen as practical or desirable by civil servants. They are sympathetic to their minister's political aims, indeed many ministers – such as Jack Straw – started their political careers as special advisers. When Barbara Castle was Secretary of State for Social Services, she had two advisers: Brian Abel-Smith, a Professor at the London School of Economics (who had provided advice for the Guillebaud Committee in the 1950s, see chapter 1), and Jack Straw. The Thatcher Government's use of Sir Roy Griffiths, an industrialist, as a source of radical advice is outlined in box 2.4.

Box 2.4 Impact of special advisers: Sir Roy Griffiths and the Thatcher Government

Background Sir Roy Griffiths (1926–94) was a businessman. He was a Director of Monsanto Europe (1964–8) before moving to Sainsbury's, where he was a Director (1968–91), Deputy Chairman (1975–91) and Managing Director (1979–88).

Role as adviser In 1981 the newly appointed Secretary of State for Social Services, Sir Norman Fowler, invited Griffiths to review NHS management. Following the implementation of his recommendations, Sir Roy was invited to be Deputy Chairman of the NHS Management Board (1986–9) and NHS Policy Board (1986–94), and to be the government adviser on the NHS (1986–94).

Impact on policy Griffiths was Fowler's trusted confidant and came to be trusted by the Prime Minister, Margaret Thatcher. He played a key role in the restructuring of both health and social care in England and stimulated the development of general management in the NHS and the development of managed or internal markets in both the NHS and social care

Examples of his advice

The NHS Management Inquiry (1983) When Fowler became Secretary of State for Social Services, he was committed to Thatcherite reforms and in particular to rolling back the frontiers of the state and, in the case of the NHS, reducing its staffing and costs. His initial attempts to reduce costs were frustrated by the Regional Health Authorities, so he turned to Griffiths for advice. Griffiths agreed to chair a small inquiry team and produce a short report. In the Report, Griffiths argued that neither the NHS nor the Department of Health and Social Security were fit for purpose and both required operational and strategic management. In the NHS this was to involve the development of general management and, in the Department of Health and Social Security, supervisory and management boards. These recommendations were accepted.

Community Care Agenda for Change (1988) In the 1980s there was a rapid and unplanned expansion of social security payments for older people living in residential care. Again Fowler turned to Griffiths for advice. Griffiths reviewed the current system and suggested that local authorities should take over the management of these monies and assess the needs of older people and use the monies to meet these needs in the most cost-effective manner possible, i.e. either by providing care packages so individuals could remain at home or funding care in residential or nursing homes. The basic principles outlined by Griffiths, that local authorities should assess need and purchase services mainly from the private sector, formed the basis of the 1990 NHS and Community Care Act.

Civil servants

These are permanent and confidential advisers to ministers and key experts in policy. Ministers have a duty to consult their civil servants. The modern relationship between ministers and civil servants developed in the nineteenth century alongside the expansion of government activities. Alongside the long-established Treasury, the Home Office and Foreign Office were created in 1782, and in 1786 the Board of Trade was re-established (Hennessy 1990: 25–30). These early ministries were small, tended to have very broad remits and appointed officials on the basis of political patronage. Thus, when the Home Office was established in 1782, the Minister, the Home Secretary, was supported by thirty officials and was responsible not only for maintaining the King's peace but also for colonial affairs. Hennessy has argued that the Home Office was 'Whitehall's charlady mopping up the pools of activity that did not fit tidily into other institutional containers' (1990: 28). As government activity grew, so the Home Office was able to spin off activities to new departments. As the state's involvement in welfare expanded through Lunacy and Poor Law legislation, so the Home Office took on the oversight of the various regulatory bodies that supervised the new asylums and workhouses.

Initially there was no clear divide between the role of ministers and civil servants. For example, ministers in the early nineteenth century, such as the Foreign Secretary Castlereagh, would often ignore their officials by doing their own paperwork (Hennessy 1990: 28). The Treasury, with its oversight of public spending, was committed to developing an efficient civil service with an intellectual elite concentrating on policy making (for discussion of the reforms and their implications, see Hennessy 1990: 32–51). When William Gladstone became Chancellor of the Exchequer in 1852, he commissioned

Stafford Northcote (a politician and former civil servant) and Charles Trevelyan (the Permanent Secretary and the most senior civil servant at the Treasury) to review the civil service. The review was completed in 1854 but not fully implemented until 1870. It recommended the establishment of an elite and permanent cadre of civil servants recruited directly from the universities by competitive exam who would concentrate on the intellectual work needed to support policy making. They would delegate routine activities and the administration of services to inferior grades in the civil service. This system remains the basis of the bureaucratic machine of contemporary British government.

The creation of an elite cadre of top civil servants had implications for the relationship between ministers and civil servants. This new elite expected to be consulted about and to give their advice on policies – indeed, given their intellectual skills and knowledge, they would expect to have considerable influence over the development of policy. Thus, the Northcote–Trevelyan reforms created the British ministerial system of policy making in which ministers provide political oversight of policy and expert career civil servants offer policy advice and oversee the implementation of policy.

The Department of Health provides ministers with access to civil servants who have two complementary types of expertise: career civil servants and professional civil servants who build up their expertise through professional training and practice and are then recruited into the department.

Career civil servants have developed knowledge of health policy and the operation of government machinery in Whitehall through a career within the civil service, often within the department itself. The Permanent Secretary is the most senior career civil servant and he (until the Coalition Government appointed a woman, Una O'Brien, to the post in October 2010, it has always been a man in the Department of Health) is accountable to ministers and Parliament for the operation of the Department. Until the 1990s Permanent Secretaries were very much internal departmental appointments. For example, Sir Christopher France, who was Permanent Secretary from 1988 until 1992, started his career in the Treasury (1959–84) before moving to the Department of Health and Social Security, where he became a Deputy Secretary (1984). He was promoted to second Permanent Secretary in 1986, and Permanent Secretary in 1988.

This pattern was disrupted in 2000 when Nigel Crisp, whose background is described in box 2.5, was appointed as both

---

Box 2.5 Nigel Crisp: Permanent Secretary and NHS Chief Executive, 2000–2006

Background Nigel Crisp was born in 1952 and educated at the University of Cambridge (degree in Philosophy). He first worked in community services before moving into NHS management, progressing from a General Manager post in East Berkshire's learning disability service (1986) to the post of Chief Executive of Oxford Radcliffe Hospitals NHS Trust, one of the largest academic medical centres in the NHS. He moved into the civil service in 1997 as Regional Director for the NHS in South Thames, becoming the Director of the newly formed London Region in 1999, where his commitment to the New Labour programme of reforms was evident. In 2000 he was appointed to the combined post of the Permanent Secretary and the Chief Executive of the NHS.

Role as a civil servant In his dual role, Nigel Crisp was responsible both for providing oversight of the Department of Health and for managing the National Health Service in England. He was responsible for implementing the programme of reform announced in the White Paper *The New NHS: Modern, Dependable* (Department of Health 1997) and developed in *The NHS Plan* (Department of Health 2000a), and ensuring that the NHS and its constituent Trusts all remained within budget.

End of the experiment In the winter of 2005/6, it became clear that many NHS Trusts were seriously over budget. Crisp, as the Department's Accounting Officer accountable to Parliament for expenditure, announced his premature retirement in March 2006, acknowledging his disappointment with the current financial problems of parts of the NHS. He was elevated to the peerage as Baron Crisp of Eaglescliffe in April 2006. His post was split, with Hugh Taylor becoming Acting Permanent Secretary and Sir Ian Carruthers Acting NHS Chief Executive.

---

the Permanent Secretary and the Chief Executive of the NHS. When Nigel Crisp resigned unexpectedly in March 2007, the traditional pattern was re-established. The job was split and his successor as Permanent Secretary, Hugh Taylor, was a career civil servant.

Alongside 'career' civil servants, the Department of Health recruits professionals as civil servants. Such civil servants are not young graduates recruited directly from university and trained within the civil service but senior practitioners who have had successful professional careers. The most senior professional adviser is the Chief Medical Officer and while there are similarities between the role of the Permanent Secretary and that of the Chief Medical Officer – both effectively control the advice provided to ministers in their area of expertise – there are important differences. The Permanent Secretary line-manages the key policy directorates in the Department. The Permanent Secretary's role is based in and restricted to the Department. In contrast the Chief Medical Officer role extends beyond the Department. He or she is the principal medical adviser not only to the Secretary of State for Health but also to the Prime Minister and the whole government. The creation of the Chief Medical Office post predates both the formation of the NHS in 1948 and the formation of the Ministry of Health in 1919.

The Chief Medical Officer claims a standing as an expert who can be, when necessary, independent of government. For example, on his website the Chief Medical Officer Sir Liam Donaldson acknowledged his role as a representative of government but stressed his accountability to the public: 'I represent the Government, for which I work, the medical profession, which I try to listen to, and the public. My moral principle is that if ever there is a conflict it is the public who wins' (Donaldson 2008). This autonomy is reflected in the fact that the Chief Medical Officer can make public statements about policy, a privilege normally reserved for ministers. Thus the Chief Medical Officer can effectively make policy statements. For example, in 2009, the Chief Medical Officer (Donaldson 2010) announced that the harm caused to others by those drinking to excess should be considered and treated in the same way as the harm that smokers caused to others, i.e. as 'passive drinking', and that the Government should take action to increase the real price of alcohol to reduce consumption and harm (Burgess 2009). Given the high public profiles of CMOs, despite their scientific background they can become politically associated with a particular government. For example Sir Liam Donaldson was the Chief Medical Officer from 1998 till 2010 for nearly the whole period that the Labour Party was in government (1997–2010) and his resignation coincided with the defeat of the Labour Government in May 2010. As CMO his strong interest in risk fitted well with dominant New Labour ideology and he became closely associated with the New Labour programme of health reforms (we discuss the ideology underpinning this programme of reforms in chapter 8). The incoming Coalition Government appointed Dame Sally Davies as Interim CMO, making the appointment permanent in March 2011. This appointment represented a major shift in emphasis. Dame Sally Davies was not a public health doctor. Her background was in scientific research, indeed she was Director General of the NHS Research and Development programme and Chief Scientific Adviser for the Department of Health and the NHS (Department of Health 2011b).

The importance of both career civil servants and professionals in providing the knowledge required in health policy making raises the issue of how the types of expert and expertise relate to each other, and we will focus on this in the final section of this chapter.

2.5 Expertise in health policy making: generic and professional experts

Given the complexity of health issues, 'rational' health policy making needs to draw on generic knowledge, for example how complex organisational systems such as hospitals can be most effectively organised, as well as more specialist knowledge about the nature of specific diseases and the best way of managing them.

The post-war reliance on generic expertise

As we noted in chapter 1, when the NHS was set up in 1948 the main emphasis was on running the system within the resources provided. Thus the emphasis was on generic expertise and the organisation of the Ministry of Health was based on, and reflected, the main parts of the service – with separate groups of civil servants dealing with the services provided by local authorities, regional hospital boards and executive councils that contracted for primary care services such as general practice. There was initially little perceived need for specialist expertise and knowledge. The Ministry of Health did have a Chief Medical Officer but since the scope of public health was limited this curtailed his influence. The Ministry only increased its specialist expertise slowly. For example the Ministry of Health appointed its first statistician in 1955 in response to parliamentary criticism (Brown and Steele 1979: 250). In the immediate post-war period most specialist advice tended to come from professional bodies such as the British Medical Association, which was effectively co-opted into the policy-making process, as we noted in chapter 1.

The expansion of professional expertise and its integration into a policy-making machine: the 1971 reform of the Department of Health and Social Security

We noted in chapter 1 that the scope of health policy making expanded in the 1960s, and with it the demand for more specialist knowledge. In 1970, Sir Keith Joseph as the new Conservative Secretary of State decided to reform the system of health policy making, in preparation for the restructuring of the system of delivering health that took place in 1974. Both reforms drew on private-sector managerial consultants such as McKinsey's and both had similar features: rational planning and management systems based on multidisciplinary teams bringing together the knowledge of generalists and health professionals.

Under the 1971 restructuring of the Department of Health and Social Security, the new system was designed to effectively manage policy by developing an overall long-term strategy based on expert professional advice and ensuring it shaped the development of the NHS through a planning process. This was effectively linked to the allocation of resources, as shown in figure 2.4. At the heart of the system were multidisciplinary teams. The teams in the Policy Group focused on the needs of specific clients, such as children or people with mental illness. They brought together professionals (doctors, nurses, social workers) and generalist civil servants. Their role was to amass evidence on the most effective ways of providing care and to issue guidance to the NHS and social services departments on best practice. These teams were responsible for the series of policy statements we mentioned in chapter 1, e.g. *Better Services for the Mentally Ill* (Department of Health and Social Security 1975), *A Happier Old Age* (Department of Health and Social Security 1978), *Drinking Sensibly* (Department of Health and Social Security 1981). These policy teams also provided evidence to a Departmental Policy Planning Unit on the resources which would be needed to achieve desired changes and standards. This Unit advised Ministers on the ways in which resources should be allocated to achieve government priorities, and from 1976 ministerial decisions on resource allocation were issued as guidance on priorities as described in box 2.6.

An aim of this new system was to integrate policy making with the implementation of policy, i.e. the delivery of health and social care. At the local level (Area Health Authorities and co-terminous social

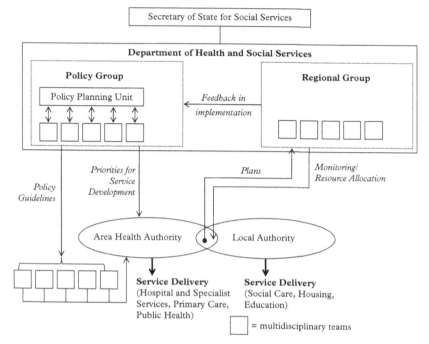

Figure 2.4   Department of Health and Social Security – Managing and Planning a Health Care System (post 1971)

services departments), joint care planning teams mirrored the policy-making groups in the Department. They were both multidisciplinary teams with responsibility for specific client groups. The local teams were expected to use national guidance to develop long- and short-term local plans to implement government policy. These plans were then submitted to the Regional Group of the Department in which multidisciplinary groups would check them against the guidance, allocate the resources to achieve them, monitor progress against plans, and feedback to the Policy Planning Unit on any problems in implementation.

Developing strategic leadership in health policy

The early 1970s reforms of the Department of Health and Social Security, the NHS and local authority services created an elegant rational policy-making machine. The priority-setting exercise was designed to set the overall context, framework or 'direction of travel' of the NHS and related services, while client group teams were meant

---

Box 2.6   Managerialism and policy making: developing priorities in the mid-1970s

Historical context   Despite various economic and financial crises and social tension, Ministers and senior civil servants pushed ahead with the reforms of health and social care and initiated the new policy-making and planning system in the mid-1970s.

Participants   In the department, multidisciplinary groups focused on the needs of specific client groups, sought funding for the development of new patterns of service, submitting proposed developments to a departmental Policy Planning Unit.

Process   The Policy Planning Unit considered the resources available and ministerial wishes and developed an overall set of priorities designed to inform allocation to and development of local services.

Policy outcomes   The first of a series of documents on priorities was issued in 1976 (Department of Health and Social Security 1976a) and indicated that deprived 'Cinderella services' – especially services for older people, and people with mental illness or learning disabilities – should receive additional funds. Services for other adults were to operate within existing budgets, while funding for maternity services were to be reduced in line with reductions in the birth rate.

---

to provide the detailed policies to inform the local plans for specific services.

Unfortunately, the timing of the reforms was poor. They coincided with a major economic crisis during which the Labour Government lost control of public expenditure and then introduced cash limits to restrain it. By 1979 when the Conservatives, led by Margaret Thatcher, returned to power, public expenditure, rational planning and the welfare professions that benefited from both were out of favour. Thatcher expected her ministers to implement a programme of radical reform. Thus Sir Norman Fowler entitled his account of his period in government, including being Secretary of State for Social Services, *Ministers Decide* (1991). However, as we noted earlier in this chapter (see box 2.4), Fowler was frustrated by the complex system of policy making dominated by the detailed work of multidisciplinary teams. He instigated reform of the Department to ensure that the ministers could control the overall direction of policy. Thus, at the centre of current policy making is a strategic Departmental Board with an emphasis on generic expertise to ensure that there is clear policy direction through the Board: 'The Departmental Board forms the strategic and operational leadership of the department. It brings together our ministerial team, our civil service leaders and a strengthened network of non-executives, recruited from outside Government' (Department of Health 2011c).

The main concern of the Board is the development of policies that will ensure the efficient management and delivery of health and social care services. The Coalition Government notes that 'Ministers work with the Departmental board and clinical specialists to ensure the Department meets its objectives' (Department of Health 2011c) and defines the functions of the Board in the following way:

> The Departmental Board forms the collective strategic and operational leadership of the Department. Its remit is performance and delivery, including appropriate oversight of sponsored bodies. The Departmental Board is responsible for:
>
> • supporting Ministers on strategic issues linked to the development and implementation of the Government's objectives for the health and social care system,
> • ensuring there is strategic alignment across the bodies accountable to Department of Health for the health and care system,
> • agreeing the department's three-year rolling business plan,
> • ensuring the sound financial management of the department, in the context of the business plan,
> • oversight of progress against business plan milestones, including performance against efficiency metrics,
> • assurance on performance of the department's sponsored bodies, and
> • (on advice from the Executive Board) ensuring effective management of risks within the department and its sponsored bodies. (Department of Health 2011d)

The Board is chaired by the Secretary of State and includes all the ministers and four non-Executive members (Department of Health 2011d) to give the Board access to independent and critical expertise and to 'challenge the quality of the policy formulation process' (Department of Health 2008b). The Board does include the five top civil servants in the department but only one of these comes from a health professional background – the Chief Medical Officer – the others, such as the Permanent Secretary, are career civil servants.

The Board can be seen as an important part of the rational policy-making process. It ensures that ministers can access expertise on key policy issues and it can see the big picture, the major problems and issues, and direct policy strategies to meeting these issues. However, given the wide scope of departmental policies, the Board cannot provide detailed advice on specific issues and is supplemented by individuals and groups focusing on the details of such issues.

Fulfilling the Enlightenment dream: grounding decisions in an Encyclopaedia of scientific knowledge

While the 1971 reform of the Department of Health and Social Security relied on multidisciplinary groups to provide policy advice about specific client groups, there has been increasing emphasis on the scientific codification of evidence and the development of guidelines based on these frameworks. In some ways this can be seen as the fulfilment of the Enlightenment dream, the creation of a document that synthesises all the scientific knowledge available as the basis for rational decision making.

There has been substantial investment in a range of activities underpinning the development of this Encyclopaedia of knowledge about health and health care. For example, in 1992, the first Director of the NHS Research and Development approved funding of 'a Cochrane Centre' 'to facilitate the preparation of systematic reviews of randomised controlled trials of health care' (Cochrane Collaboration 2011). A key element in this development has been the appointment of senior professionals as National Clinical Directors or 'Tsars' for specific diseases or client groups. In 2011 there were sixteen Directors including:

- Professor Roger Boyle, National Director for Heart Disease and Stroke
- Professor Louis Appleby, formerly National Director for Mental Health then National Clinical Director for Health and Criminal Justice
- Professor Mike Richards, National Clinical Director for Cancer

These Directors have a central role to play in the development and implementation of rational policies in their area of responsibility.

> **Box 2.7 Development of the 2005 Cancer Framework (Expert Advisory Group on Cancer 2005)**
>
> *Context* There was concern in the Department of Health and the media that survival rates for cancer treatment in the UK lagged behind those in other developed countries.
>
> *Process* The Chief Medical Officers for England (Sir Kenneth Calman) and Wales (Dame Deidre Hine) commissioned and chaired a working party of fourteen cancer experts. The working party reviewed current evidence where it was available, and used an expert consensus where there was no firm evidence base.
>
> *Policy outcome* The working group recommended guidelines for the development of cancer services in the UK. These guidelines were then issued by the Department of Health and formed the basis of the provision of local services, and standards against which local clinicians could judge effectiveness.

In each area, expert groups codify the best available knowledge or evidence into National Service Frameworks or strategies. These evidence-based strategies 'set clear requirements for care' (National Health Service 2010) for each client or disease area and provide the basis for developing and monitoring services: 'National clinical directors and advisors – sometimes referred to as Tsars – are experts that oversee the implementation of a national service framework (NSF) or major clinical or service strategy. They act as advocates for the NSFs or strategy within the NHS and other services, and represent the NHS and other services in the Department of Health' (Department of Health 2010d).

The first Framework was one for Cancer created in 2005, and the Chief Medical Officers in England and Wales took the lead in establishing the expert working group which synthesised existing evidence on the most effective cancer services (see box 2.7). By 2008 there were ten Frameworks (National Health Service 2010).

While expert working parties remain an important part of the process of developing Frameworks, they are complemented by a new organisation, the National Institute for Health and Clinical Excellence (NICE). This is an 'arm's-length' organisation, i.e. funded by the Government but operating independently to enhance the legitimacy of its findings. It is designed to access and summarise

---

Box 2.8   Rational policy making: the case of Herceptin (Trastuzumab) and breast cancer

Historical context   Herceptin was a new drug developed by an American drug company that was used alongside surgery and chemotherapy to treat breast cancer. The drug company claimed it substantially reduced mortality from breast cancer, especially of women with the more aggressive HER2 form of breast cancer.

Process   NICE commissioned a 'rapid and systematic review of clinical effectiveness and cost-effectiveness' from a team of researchers at the University of York. The team reviewed existing published (plus confidential) evidence from clinical trials and economic evaluations. This review of evidence found that Herceptin reduced mortality but increased the costs of treatment and that each Life Year Gained cost £14,069, but due to side-effects of the treatment each QALY costs £29,448.

Policy outcomes   NICE issued guidance recommending that Health Commissioners should fund Herceptin treatment for women with HER2 breast cancer.

---

the evidence on current practice, providing guidance on current *best practice*. It produces guidance in three main areas of health:

- public health – guidance on the promotion of good health and the prevention of ill health, for those working in the NHS, local authorities and the wider public and voluntary sector
- health technologies – guidance on the use of new and existing medicines, treatments and procedures within the NHS
- clinical practice – guidance on the appropriate treatment and care of people with specific diseases and conditions within the NHS (NICE 2008a).

One aspect of NICE's work has attracted particular public and media interest and controversy – the evaluation of new technologies, such as new drugs for treating cancer. In this area NICE has sought to establish agreed objective measures for assessing the benefit of new treatments and for making recommendations for NHS funding of a new treatment. As we note in box 2.8, in the case study of the approval of Herceptin NICE used QALYs (Quality Adjusted Life

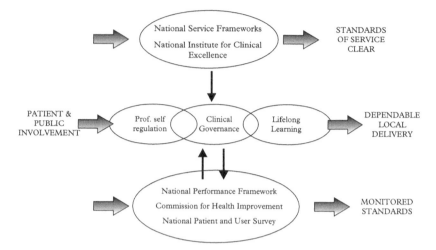

Figure 2.5   The rational system of managing health care in England
(Department of Health 1998b)

Years) (see chapter 1 box 1.2). This is a highly emotive area in which there have been public and media debates about values and allocation of scarce resources. We will return to and reconsider this case in chapters 6 and 7 (see box 7.3).

The National Clinical Directors, NICE and the National Service Framework can be seen as an expert-based system for making health policy in specific clinical areas by identifying, collating and disseminating the best knowledge or evidence about clinical practice. They form part of an overall rational system of policy making. Key elements in the overall framework (see figure 2.5) are using this knowledge to create 'dependable local delivery' of services and externally monitoring local services to ensure that they meet the specified standards.

Comment

Instrumentally rational policy making should be based on comprehensive knowledge of policy ends and the best means of achieving them. However, in the British system ministers who are key policy makers usually do not necessarily have a strong interest in or knowledge of the policies area for which they are responsible. They use confidential advisers to overcome this knowledge deficit. As the scope and complexity of health and related policy making have

expanded since 1948, so has the sophistication of the supporting
advisory system enabling the health ministers, especially in England,
to provide overall strategic leadership and, at the same time, to draw
on detailed technical and professional expertise.

KEY POINTS

• Policy making which is instrumentally rational should be grounded
  in knowledge of both policy ends and the means of achieving them,
  and requires the application of reason to define best ends and
  evaluate the benefits and costs of alternative means of achieving
  such ends.
• Ministers with formal and public responsibility for public policy
  making are selected for their political background and expertise,
  and only exceptionally do they have prior interest in and knowledge of the policy areas that they are given responsibility for.
• Ministers can and do bring in 'trusted' experts as special advisers
  to provide them with advice. Labour health ministers have tended
  to draw on academic experts, while Conservative ministers tend to
  look to the private sector.
• Health ministers have access to senior civil servants who have
  accumulated substantial administrative expertise and specialist
  knowledge during their careers, which usually have been within
  Whitehall and mainly within the area of health. In the Department
  of Health, ministers look to their senior civil service for advice and
  policies that will ensure the efficient management and delivery of
  health and social care services.
• Health ministers access professional expertise in different ways.
  They appoint senior professionals to civil servant posts within the
  Department of Health and, as in the case of the Chief Medical
  Officer, give these professionals responsibilities for advising on
  the ways in which services can and should be delivered. They
  access their expertise as part-time advisers – e.g. National Clinical
  Directors – or as members of expert working parties. They have
  set up arm's-length bodies such as NICE that commission expert
  reviews of evidence and provide guidance on the best and most
  cost-effective modes of clinical practice.
• While the scope of health policy since 1948 has remained relatively constant, the complexity has increased substantially. This
  complexity has been matched by the increased sophistication of
  the policy-making system, combining the expertise of generic civil

servants with that of health professionals. These systems can be seen as creating rational policies based on the synthesis of scientific knowledge and expert opinion.

- Current health policy making can be seen as rational in that it combines mechanisms for identifying the broad picture and setting overall strategy with systems for synthesising scientific knowledge in specific areas using these as the basis for decision making.

3

The competition for money and the limits of instrumental rationality

AIMS

To examine the importance of money in the policy-making process and consider the ways in which the objective measurability of money facilities rationality. To examine the ways in which the systems of allocating money to policies have developed in attempts to enhance efficiency and quality of outcomes.

OBJECTIVES

- To consider the role of money as a key resource in policy making and as the rational basis of health policy
- To examine the theories about the ways money is, and should be, allocated to policies and consider the influence of rationality within different forms of allocation
- To discuss the development of systems of financial resource allocation within UK government
- To examine the rationality of the current system of allocating money to health policy.

In chapters 1 and 2 we have concentrated on policy making as a process of thinking about and deciding on issues, especially identifying major social and health issues, evaluating the best way of dealing with such issues and deciding on the best course of action. However, to convert decisions into actions requires resources and without them policy making is merely an exercise in wishful thinking. In this chapter we focus on money as the key resource in policy making and consider the rationality of its allocation to health and related policies.

3.1 Money as a key resource and means of achieving rationality in policy making

Resources and policy making

Gustafsson (1983) has argued that the diffusion of power in modern society means that policy makers often cannot effectively control and guarantee appropriate resources. Thus, many policies are symbolic or pseudo-policies which are not intended to, are unlikely to or cannot be implemented.

In the United Kingdom the government protects against the danger of symbolic policy making by linking policies to resources in programmes. The term 'programme' can be used to refer either to a broad package of policies and resources, such as the Health and Personal Social Services (HPSS) programme in England, or to a narrower more focused area, such as the hospital building programme. Such programmes are characterised by their policy objectives – in the case of HPSS, improving the health of the nation, and in the case of the hospital building programme, building hospitals that are fit for purpose – as well as the resources included, e.g. in the HPSS programme the money to pay for staff and health-care facilities, and in the hospital building programme the money that will be invested in the construction of new hospitals.

While setting objectives and allocating resources to meet these objectives should be integrated, in practice they involve different relationships and processes. Individual ministers with their policy advisers take the lead in identifying policy objectives and deciding how to achieve them, and this is very much a departmental process. Ministers tend to focus on their own policy issues and have neither the time nor the inclination to be involved or interfere in the issues dealt with by their ministerial colleagues, even though the Cabinet, a committee of senior ministers chaired by the Prime Minister, should have the final say. Resources are limited so their allocation involves interaction between ministers as they compete over the funds, seeking to maximise their own share.

While money is not the only resource that governments use to achieve their objectives, it is the most important as it is a flexible resource which can be used in a variety of ways. It can be used:

- for direct payments so individuals can purchase their own services
- to purchase goods or service from a third party on behalf of service users
- to pay staff employed by a government agency to provide a service
- to invest in new facilities such as buildings and equipment.

Money is an effective medium for rational decision making. It is a constant medium of exchange that can be used for calculation and comparisons. As Weber noted, the development of the rational approach is based on the knowledge or belief that everything can be understood and mastered through calculations (Weber 1947: 139). Indeed, the scientific method that underpins the Enlightenment programme is based on quantification, the measurement of the extent of phenomena, rather than assessment of their intrinsic qualities. While it is inherently difficult to measure and compare the outcomes and benefits of different policy programmes – how does one compare the benefits of a new aircraft carrier versus those of a new MRI scanner? – it is relatively easy to compare how much they cost. Money provides a medium of control and comparison. It can be used to control the future (through budget setting), manage the present (by controlling expenditure over defined periods, usually a year) and evaluate the past (through an audit of expenditure).

Money and rationality

Money should provide the ideal mechanism for achieving 'economic' rationality in policy, 'the most efficient use of resources amongst competing ends' (Gregory 1993: 213) as it provides policy makers with a mechanism controlling the input of resources. However, there is considerable debate amongst commentators on the extent to which the allocation of money in public services can or should be rational.

Full rationality implies that resources are used in the most efficient and effective manner possible. A major source of 'irrationality' in policy making comes from institutional inertia: once a decision has been made to allocate money to a certain activity, this allocation may continue regardless of changed circumstances or the benefits generated. Therefore, decisions and the associated allocation of resources can only be rational if decision makers regularly review and reconsider past decisions. To be rational, policy makers should periodically start with a clean sheet and consider the objectives they wish to achieve and the best way of using money to attain these. This approach is often referred to as zero-based budgeting: 'an approach to budgeting that starts from the premise that no costs or activities should be factored into the plans for the coming budget period, just because they figured in the costs or activities for the current or previous periods. Rather, everything that is to be included in the budget must be considered and justified' (CIPFA 2006: 1). Thus, zero-based budgeting is designed to create the instrumental rational link between means (money) and ends (policy objectives). It seeks to break an overall programme of activity into discrete parts, or decision packages, and then subject each part to a thorough analysis to identify the most efficient way of achieving the desired objectives in that area (Lewis 2006: 1).

The Treasury claimed to use this approach in 1998 when planning expenditure allocations for government activities in the UK: 'The 1998 Comprehensive Spending Review (CSR), which was published in July 1998, was a comprehensive review of departmental aims and objectives alongside a zero-based analysis of each spending programme to determine the best way of delivering the Government's objectives' (Her Majesty's Treasury 1998). The advocates of zero-based budgeting note that the world in which policy decisions have to be made is not perfect. Obtaining comprehensive information is time-consuming and costly. As the Chartered Institute of Public Finance and Accountancy noted in its briefing document on zero-based budgeting: 'This [zero-based budgeting] initially appears to be a very resource hungry approach, and if applied in this simplistic form, would quickly fall foul of the law of diminishing returns' (CIPFA 2006: 1).

This difficulty can be dealt with by limiting the scope of review and seeking 'bounded' rather than 'full' rationality – or, in CIPFA's terms, 'the application of practical common sense' (2006: 1). However, there is a further, more fundamental caveat: much of the required knowledge is about the future, and the future is uncertain and difficult to predict. For example, as we note in box 3.1, when the Treasury invited Sir Derek Wanless to predict the future cost of funding the NHS he produced three separate estimates of likely future expenditure.

Economists such as Keynes have argued that, because of the imperfections of the real world, decision making cannot be rational and, in the absence of appropriate knowledge, individuals have to fall back on 'irrationality' as the basis of decision making:

> human decisions affecting the future, whether personal or political or
> economic, cannot depend on strict mathematical expectation, since

Box 3.1   Predicting the future cost of the NHS: The Wanless Report (Wanless 2002)

Historical context   In March 2001 the Chancellor of the Exchequer, Gordon Brown, invited Sir Derek Wanless, a banker, to undertake a review of the long-term trends affecting the health service in the United Kingdom over the next twenty years. Wanless stated that he had been asked to quantify *'the financial and other resources required to ensure that the NHS can provide a publicly funded, comprehensive, high quality service available on the basis of clinical need and not ability to pay'* (Letter to the Chancellor of the Exchequer, in Wanless 2002). In undertaking his review, Sir Derek Wanless was supported by the Health Trends Review team in the Treasury and also commissioned research on the health trends and costs in eight other countries.

Key areas of uncertainty   The final report of the review identified various areas of uncertainty, including the willingness of individuals to accept public health advice and take responsibility for their own health, and the ability of the NHS to make the best use of technology and resources. The review presented three scenarios:
* scenario 1: *solid progress* – people become more engaged in managing their health. The health service is responsive, takes up new technology and uses resources more efficiently;
* scenario 2: *slow uptake* – there is no change in the level of people's involvement in managing their own health. The health service is relatively unresponsive to change with low rates of technology uptake and low productivity;
* scenario 3: *fully engaged* – the level of people's involvement in managing their own health is high. The health service is responsive to change with high take-up of technology especially to prevent disease, and uses resources more efficiently.

Predictions   The three scenarios were linked to three different cost predictions. The review predicted that the best results in terms of costs and outcomes, especially increased life expectancy, would be in the fully engaged scenario. While the health ministers and the departments could control some factors, such as the efficiency with which the NHS used resources, other factors, such as individuals' willingness to be engaged in proactive management of their health, were more difficult to influence.

Table 3.1   Total NHS spending (£ billions, 2002–3 prices)

Years	2002–3	2007–8	2012–13	2017–18	2022–3
Solid progress	68	96	121	141	161
Slow uptake	68	97	127	155	184
Fully engaged	68	96	119	137	154

(*Source:*   Wanless 2002)

the basis for making such calculations does not exist; and that it is our innate urge to activity which makes the wheels go round, our rational selves choosing between the alternatives as best we are able, calculating where we can, but often falling back for our motive on whim or sentiment or chance. (Keynes 1973: 162–3)

Simon (1976) sought to reframe rationality to deal with the imperfections of the real world. He defined rationality in terms of means and ends and selecting the best means to achieve the desired ends. In budgeting, this means either selecting the course of action that offers the most desirable outcome or selecting the most cost-effective method of achieving a specified outcome (1976: 39). Simon acknowledged the intrinsic uncertainty underpinning decision making, especially the incompleteness of knowledge. As a result, he argued that decision makers have to limit uncertainty: 'It is obviously impossible for the individual to know all his alternatives and all their consequences, and this impossibility is a very important departure of actual behaviour from the model of objective rationality' (Simon 1976: 67).

Since decision makers cannot achieve maximum benefits, they should maximise benefits within the limits of current constraints. Thus, rationality is limited or bounded by practical constraints. In such circumstances, those making decisions should aim 'for a course of action that is satisfactory or "good enough"' (Simon 1976: xxix). Such 'satisficing' involves identifying the most important objectives and using resources to achieve these objectives rather than considering all possible outcomes. It is 'good enough' and is a product of the practical constraints of individuals dealing with complex problems in an uncertain world. He suggested that individuals '*satisfice* because they do not have the wits to *maximize*' (Simon 1976: xxvii, italics in the original).

For Simon, rationality is an important objective, something that should be strived for but can never be fully achieved. However, Lindblom has argued that such an approach is idealistic and that decision-makers should concentrate on immediate problems and issues rather than trying to create some ideal future state. Thus, for Lindblom, full rationality is neither a good description of the reality of decision making and resource allocation in government agency, nor is it a particularly desirable approach to such decisions.

Lindblom (1959) noted that administrators in public services do not start with a clean sheet but from the basis of existing services and funding. They concentrate on likely changes at the margin, the probable increases or reduction in funding. In Lindblom's view, this approach is cost-effective. It maximises the use of scarce resources including time and knowledge, and avoids wastage or conflict. Thus incrementalism is rational in that it makes effective use of time, focusing on realistic ways of improving outcomes:

> Since policy analysis is incremental, exploratory, serial, and marked by adjustments of ends to means it is expected that stable long-term aspirations will not appear as dominant critical values in the eyes of the analyst. The characteristics of strategy support and encourage the analyst to identify situations or ills from which to move *away* rather than goals *towards* which to move. (Braybrooke and Lindblom 1963: 102, italics in the original)

While advocates of rational policy making acknowledge that Lindblom's model captures some of the reality of policy making, they argue that incrementalism does not encourage policy makers to critically reflect on or challenge previous decisions and allocations. It effectively maintains and builds on the status quo. As Dror noted, 'The "rational-comprehensive" model has at least the advantage of stimulating administrators to get a little outside their regular routine, while Lindblom's model justifies a policy of "no effort". Taken together, the limited validity of the "muddling through" thesis and its inertia-reinforcing implications constitute a very serious weakness' (Dror 1964: 155).

Smith and May argue that the rationality/incrementalism dichotomy is a false one and that it is possible to combine them, using incrementalism to deal with immediate problems and issues and rationality to identify emerging issues and important changes that will effect policy in the long term. They argue that the two approaches can be combined in *mixed scanning* which has two linked phases of decision making: 'Initially a broad sweep is made of policy options and these are assessed against stated values in general terms. Then, within this framework, decision making proceeds incrementally in matters of detail' (Smith and May 1993: 202).

It is clear that commentators who seek to analyse the ways in which policy makers allocate resources to policies accept that rationality is important in such decision making. However, it is also evident that they define rationality differently. In the remainder of this chapter we will examine the nature of rationality within resource allocation in the UK.

3.2 Allocating public expenditure in the UK: a search for rationality and control

The Impact of the welfare state on the management of public finances

Until the Second World War, the Treasury and its chief minister, the Chancellor of the Exchequer, were first and foremost the government's banker and were responsible for balancing the books by ensuring that the income raised through taxation was sufficient to cover ministerial spending commitments. As part of the welfare reforms stemming from the 1942 Beveridge Report, post-war Chancellors and the Treasury accepted an expanded role. To avoid the errors that converted the financial collapse of the American Stock Exchange in 1929 into the global Depression of the 1930s (with its major social and political consequences), the Treasury accepted responsibility for managing the economy to sustain demand and employment.

In the 1930s, Keynes noted that the 'outstanding faults of the economic society in which we live are its failure to provide for full employment and its arbitrary and inequitable distribution of wealth and incomes' (1973: 372). He had argued that the government could and should intervene in the economy in order to sustain demand to ensure the full use of available resources, but that such intervention would not essentially modify the operation of the capitalist market economy: 'For if effective demand is deficient, not only is the public scandal of wasted resources intolerable, but the individual enterpriser who seeks to bring these resources into action is operating with the odds loaded against him' (Keynes 1973: 380–1).

The adoption of Keynes's ideas widened the scope of Treasury activities. It also undermined the direct link between government income and expenditure which pre-war Chancellors and the Treasury used to control spending ministers and their departments. Keynes argued that governments should operate in a counter-intuitive way. During recessions, when the aggregate demand in the economy fell, the government should increase expenditure to sustain demand and ensure full use of economic resources, including full employment of human resources. In such circumstances the government would incur a deficit (due to lower tax revenues and higher expenditure) which would be paid back when the recession ended. Gordon Brown, as Chancellor of the Exchequer (1997–2007), adopted the so-called 'golden rule' (Her Majesty's Treasury 1998) that specified that over an economic cycle the government should balance the budget and only borrow to invest (Her Majesty's Treasury 2005).

As Heclo and Wildavsky (1981: 204) noted, in the immediate post-war period Chancellors and the Treasury found it difficult to deal with their expanded and changed role. The new role of managing the economy tended to take precedence. Spending was popular and the Treasury felt that 'forceful spending ministers were able to push through their programmes, willy nilly, and with little thought for the morrow. The Chancellor and the Treasury seemed to have lost authority' (Heclo and Wildavsky 1981: 204).

Treasury attempts to instigate reviews of welfare spending, such as the Guillebaud Review of the costs of the NHS which we discussed in chapter 1, tended to backfire, leading to calls for more spending. When the Chancellor did try to take a hard line, as with proposals to introduce prescription charges to control demand for NHS services, there were high political costs, as we show in box 3.2.

Despite such highly visible difficulties, in the early 1950s the Treasury was actually rather successful in restraining public expenditure. The Guillebaud Committee commissioned a study of health spending which showed that expenditure on the NHS, as a proportion of Gross National Product, had fallen from 3.75 per cent in 1949/50 to 3.24 per cent in 1953/4. However, this fall masked fluctuations and the 1950s were characterised by annual conflicts over public expenditure, creating a 'stop–go' economy (*Oxford Dictionary of Economics* n.d.), 'stop' when the Treasury imposed a reduction, and 'go' when the Treasury allowed demand to increase and spending ministers to increase their spending. As Heclo and Wildavsky noted, this not only had negative effects for the Government (undermining spending plans) but had knock-on effects for the private sector, creating fluctuating demand (1981: xxvii).

The tension over spending culminated in a political test of will between the Chancellor and spending ministers in 1957. In response to a sterling crisis, the Chancellor, Thorneycroft, sought to introduce a series of expenditure cuts. The Cabinet rejected his proposal to cut expenditure by '£50m, a small but symbolic amount' (Hennessy

---

Box 3.2   Controlling health expenditure: the case of prescription charges

Context   Given the lack of information about costs of existing health care, the initial costs of the NHS in 1948 and 1949 substantially exceeded the spending allocation approved by Parliament. There were unplanned increases in funding during a period of austerity. Despite health ministers' optimism that, following the initial start-up, costs would fall, the Chancellor and Treasury were concerned about the impact of rising health expenditure. While pressure on costs came from a number of sources, including staff pay and running the new hospital service, there was evidence of increased demand-led expenditure such as spending on drugs, spectacles and dentures dispensed in the community.

Process   There was a lack of information and the main protagonists took ideological stances. Nye Bevan (Minister of Health) was committed to a 'socialist' NHS free at the point of access, whereas the Chancellor, Sir Stafford Cripps, and his successor Hugh Gaitskell were committed to pragmatic control of public expenditure and ensuring that an expanding health service offered counterbalancing savings. The policy developed through internal dialogue and conflict between senior ministers. In 1950 a compromise solution was reached, with Bevan agreeing to the creation of a cabinet committee to oversee NHS spending, plus a ceiling on health expenditure of £393 million for 1950/1 and Cripps reserving the right to introduce prescription charges if this ceiling was broken. When Bevan was replaced by Marquand at the end of 1950, the new minister was more flexible, agreeing to Gaitskell's proposal for cost-cutting measures including prescription charges.

Policy outcome   In his April 1951 budget, Gaitskell announced a modest charge in respect of some dental and optical services. In April 1951 a bill was introduced in the Commons to provide legal authority for charges and this received Royal Assent in May as the 1951 NHS Amendment Act. There was a major political fall-out from this new policy, with the resignation of senior left-wing ministers including Nye Bevan and Harold Wilson. The weakened Government called a general election in October 1951 to seek a new mandate. They lost the election and the Labour Party did not regain power until 1964.

1990: 178), and the Chancellor and his two junior colleagues (including Enoch Powell who was subsequently to become Minister of Health) resigned in January 1958. In accepting his resignation, the Prime Minister, Harold Macmillan, signalled the commitment of the Conservative Government to the welfare state, arguing that in modern society the government had 'an inescapable obligation to large sections of the community – the evasion of which would be both inequitable and unacceptable to public opinion' (cited in Lowe 1997: 466).

Developing a more rational system of allocating public expenditure: PESC

The Treasury's reluctant acceptance that the welfare state was here to stay resulted in major changes, and the relatively ad hoc system of allocating expenditure was replaced by a more systematic approach grounded in a restructuring of the Treasury and the development of a new system for planning expenditure.

The Treasury was restructured into three new Groups (Lowe 1997: 466) reflecting its major responsibilities and functions:

- Public Sector Group responsible for government spending
- National Economy Group responsible for demand management
- Finance Group responsible for monetary policy and international finance.

In 1961, the Prime Minister, Harold Macmillan, aligned the Treasury Ministers to this new structure, giving the Chancellor of the Exchequer the lead on economic management, and creating a new Cabinet-rank post, the Chief Secretary to the Treasury, to take responsibility for government spending (Hennessy 1990: 176 and 179).

In 1958 a House of Commons Select Committee had criticised the then-current system of expenditure. Its criticism suggested the system could not be considered rational as the cost of programmes was not properly estimated, resulting in regular additional allocations or Supplementary Estimates (Lowe 1997: 468). In response the Government appointed a committee to review expenditure. The Committee, chaired by Lord Plowden, recommended the development of a new system which reconciled the Treasury's need for control with the spending departments' desire for planning. The key recommendation of the Committee was that individual expenditure decisions should be made within the context of overall spending plans and available resources. Sir Leo Pliatzky, a senior civil servant, summarised the approach in the following way: 'that arrangements should be introduced for making surveys of public expenditure for a period of years ahead, and that all major individual decisions involving future expenditure should be taken against the background of such a survey and in relation to prospective resources' (cited in Hennessy 1990: 179).

This system is usually referred to as the PESC (Public Expenditure Survey Committee) system. Its key features included:

- an annual planning cycle so that all programmes were considered, and spending decisions made, in the same time frame;
- a projection over a five-year period of the expenditure of current programmes through the PESC survey of current policies and the factors affecting their costs;
- decisions about overall changes in expenditure and changes in specific programmes over five years were to be agreed by all ministers through the Cabinet (Thain and Wright 1995: 34).

The PESC system was substantially more rational than the previous ad hoc system of allocation. Indeed Heclo and Wildavsky argued that PESC was a major innovation in the machinery of decision making, suggesting that it 'is the most important innovation in its field in any Western nation' (1974: lxvii). The key elements of rationality in the system were its comprehensiveness and its grounding of decisions about allocations in predictions of the future and the availability of resources.

The annual cycle was comprehensive. It provided a framework in which all spending programmes could be compared. The PESC system meant that Treasury officials could overcome the limitations of their expertise by engaging civil servants from the spending departments. The prediction of future spending on existing policies was a complex exercise, and in box 3.3 we identify some of the major factors which influence costs.

While the PESC system may have been an improvement over the previous ad hoc system, it is difficult to describe it as a rational system in the sense of zero-base budgeting. There was, for example, no built-in review of past expenditure, no serious attempt to match resources to policy objectives and intended outcomes, and no attempt to maximise the benefits of public expenditure. Furthermore, even the technical aspects such as estimating the

Box 3.3   Predicting the future costs of major programmes: identifying key factors

The characteristics of different programmes, especially the nature of their policy objectives, influence the ways in which programme costs are likely to change.

The social protection programme   This involves providing income support for individuals with short-term needs – e.g. job seeker's allowance for unemployed adults – or longer-term needs, such as pensions for older people. If the policy is fixed in terms of level of benefits, then the costs will be driven by the number of claimants. In the case of job seeker's allowances, this will be influenced by the level of unemployment, and in the case of pensions, by demographic factors such as the number of older people.

The education programme   This involves providing compulsory education for children aged five to sixteen, and pre-school and further education for children and young people who make use of these opportunities. The costs of the policies are influenced by demographic factors and the level of take-up. In the 1960s, due to the post-war 'Baby Boom' there was a rising School Roll, i.e. an increasing number of children in compulsory education, with associated increases in costs in the programmes. In the 1970s the School Roll started to fall and with it predicted costs.

The health programme   This involves the provision for the treatment of illness and disability through primary and hospital care, and prevention through public health measures. The major users of services are babies and young children and older people, so demography is a key driver of NHS costs. In the 1950s the Baby Boom and the ageing of the population increased costs and, while the birth rate fell in the 1970s, with increased life expectancies it is estimated that demographic changes increase the cost of providing care by at least 1 per cent per annum. The NHS is also committed to funding all effective treatment. There is continuous innovation in treatment through improved diagnostic equipment, treatment regimes and drug therapies. It has been estimated that such innovation adds at least another 1 per cent to health-care costs each year.

future costs of programmes were controversial. While it was possible to identify the major drivers of programmes, as we have done in box 3.3, when it came to detailed discussions of the cost projection of existing policies there was disagreement between spending departments and the Treasury 'about what each of these elements – cost, projection and existing policy – actually means' (Heclo and Wildavsky 1981: 217). Therefore, even the most rational component of the system, the cost projection, provided scope for political negotiation and bargaining. A closer look at individual programmes shows that the political context and bargains were more important than rational means–end calculations. In chapter 1 we described the 1962 Hospital Plan, emphasising its rational elements. In box 3.4, we draw out the contingent elements that shaped the development of the Plan.

Rationality in the PESC system was extremely bounded. The participants in the process sought to use the resources at their disposal – authority, finance, information, expertise and organisation – to obtain the best possible deal. This involved 'partly "balancing" and partly "optimizing"' (Thain and Wright 1995: 167) through a process of negotiation and partisan mutual adjustment:

> A strength of the PESC exercise is that it goes on year after year. Eventually most initial disagreements are negotiated and differences between the Treasury and the departments are narrowed down to more manageable proportions . . . Over the years a record of understandings about the meaning of existing policy is built up . . . For each participant, uncertainty is reduced and security increased. (Heclo and Wildavsky 1981: 220)

Thus, in the PESC system, the focus was on the relatively small increment of new spending or savings. A senior civil servant noted that 'What PESC does . . . is prevent chopping and changing policies and ensures change will be at the margins' (cited in Heclo and Wildavsky 1981: 238). It was, as Heclo and Wildavsky noted, 'incrementalism to the nth power' (1981: 238–42): 'In short, PESC has enshrined incrementalism with a vengeance . . . If PESC helps prevent departments from going beyond established bounds, it also commits the Treasury in public to keeping their expenditures going at the predicted rate. Both sides find it more difficult to depart from the historic base' (Heclo and Wildavsky 1981: 238).

Box 3.4   The 1962 Hospital Plan reconsidered: political expediency

As we noted in box 1.6 the 1962 Hospital Plan can be considered a model of economic rationality since it used evidence from expert reviews of use of hospital services to identify how and to what extent investment would enable hospital beds to be used more efficiently and effectively. However, political factors played a key role – for example, underinvestment had been evident in reviews of hospitals undertaken in the Second World War but no action was taken. In 1956 the Guillebaud Committee recommended hospital investment with no immediate effect.

Factors preventing the introduction of a hospital investment programme before 1962
- Hostility of the Treasury to welfare spending, including major investment in hospitals.
- Absence of long-term planning. Before the introduction of PESC in 1961, public expenditure allocation tended to be short-term and ad hoc.
- Lack of political will. When the Labour Government was implementing its commitment to develop a welfare state, Nye Bevan combined the post of Minister of Health with that of Minister of Housing. He saw slum clearance and house building as the main priority for the limited capital investment available.

The combination of factors in 1960/1 that facilitated the development of the 1962 Hospital Plan
- Changed attitude in government to spending. Following the defeat of the Chancellor's attempt to limit welfare spending in 1957, and the victory of the Conservatives in the 1959 general election, based on a commitment to the welfare state, the Government was committed to a programme of modernisation underpinned by increased spending.
- Long-term planning was 'in fashion'. Following the success of planning in social democracies such as France, planning was seen as a way of modernising Britain.
- Political will and knowledge. Enoch Powell was appointed Minister of Health alongside Bruce Fraser as Permanent Secretary. Both were experienced in bureaucratic politics and both were committed to major health reform. They were

essentially 'gamekeepers' turned 'poachers', having occupied
senior posts in Treasury where they had controlled welfare
expenditure. They therefore had the political will and expertise
to negotiate a long-term funding commitment from the
Treasury.

Reviewing past decisions: PAR

Two of the major weaknesses of the PESC system were the absence
of any evaluation of the effectiveness of expenditure in achieving
policy objectives (Heald 1983: 186) and any overview of policies.
The Conservative Government elected in 1970 tried to address these
deficiencies by making changes in the machinery of government, creating the Programme Analysis and Review (PAR) system to ensure
that departments had clear policy objectives and priorities, and a
Central Policy Review Staff (CPRS) to provide advice on specific
issues and policies to the Cabinet (Chapman 1997: 44). PAR was
meant to be synchronised with the annual PESC survey so that each
year a number of sub-programmes would be scrutinised – building
up over time to a comprehensive scrutiny of all policies (Heald 1983:
186).

The PAR system failed to take root and was rapidly choked by
official secrecy, so becoming irrelevant both within the civil service
and outside (Heald 1983: 187–8). PAR was intended to bring in
outside expertise, especially from business, to improve the rationality
of decision making, but did not find great support amongst ministers, Treasury officials and other civil servants. Spending ministers
were reluctant to assist the Treasury in attacking other ministers'
programmes as it might undermine their relationship and encourage retaliation. The Treasury was concerned with overall totals not
specific areas of spending, and civil servants in spending departments
viewed it as a threat (Heald 1983: 187).

The Whitehall club culture (Moran 2003), based on communal solidarity, meant that the public expenditure system tended to
'sacrifice substantive rationality (policy results) to maintaining the
communal culture' (Heclo and Wildavsky 1981: 1). However, in the
late 1970s, the inner core of this policy community, and the informal incremental system of expenditure allocation which it managed,
was challenged by the harsh reality of a major economic and public
expenditure crisis.

3.3 The development of the public spending system: control and rationality

Economic crisis and financial disaster: the failure of PESC

The 1970s were a period of economic conflict, crisis and stagflation, with falling demand (as evidenced by rising unemployment) at the same time as inflation (increases in prices) – a set of conditions that fell outside the parameters of Keynesian economics, in which inflation reflects evidence of excess, not falling, demand in the economy. Inadequate and irresponsible political responses to these challenges (Heclo and Wildavsky 1981: xviii–xxiv) meant that the economic crisis developed into a financial disaster. In 1974 and 1975 the Treasury effectively lost control of public expenditure and this contributed to the Chancellor of Exchequer being forced to seek an emergency loan from the International Monetary Fund in 1976 to protect the value of the national currency (for a discussion of the IMF Crisis, see Hickson 2005). The public and media were first alerted to the impending disaster in 1975 when Wynne Godley, an economist who advised the House of Commons Select Committee, compared the 1971 forecast for spending in 1974/5 with actual spending. The planned growth was 12 per cent, additional policy announcements added a further 3 per cent, but this did not account for the actual increase of 28.6 per cent, or an additional unannounced £5 billion in spending which became known as the missing billions (Heclo and Wildavsky 1981: xv–xvi, lii).

In 1975 the Treasury, backed by the Labour Chancellor Denis Healey and the Chief Secretary Joel Barnett, responded to the crisis with a new regime for controlling expenditure (Hennessy 1990: 252). This system involved important modifications to PESC. Rather than responding to inflation by re-pricing spending plans – one of the major factors in the 'unplanned' increase in expenditure and the missing billions – the new system involved predicting inflation and factoring it into plans by setting cash limits. If costs for any reasons rose faster, for example due to large pay awards, then spending ministers would need to make savings elsewhere in order to deliver their programme within the agreed limits.

The New Right and squeezing the public sector

This prudent approach to allocating expenditure was a precursor to a more radical reform. In 1979 a Conservative Government led by the Prime Minister Margaret Thatcher was elected. Thatcher and her 'New Right' colleagues such as Sir Keith Joseph were convinced that the disasters of the mid-1970s showed that Keynesian economics and the social democracy it underpinned had failed, and that Hayek's alternative of a minimalist state provided an attractive, more workable alternative (see discussion of these ideologies in chapter 8). The Thatcher Government's assault on the 'club culture' of British government was particularly evident in the realm of public spending (Hennessy 1990: 628–87).

The Government was committed to cutting public spending in real terms but the modified PESC failed to deliver between 1980 and 1982. Nigel Lawson, initially as a junior Treasury Minister (1979–81) and then as Chancellor (1983–9), played an important role in revamping the system. The system which developed in the early 1980s had a number of key elements:

- *Medium-Term Financial Strategy (MTFS)*, an annually updated plan which set out the macro-economic strategy based on the outlook for the economy and provided the context for public spending decisions (Thain and Wright 1995: 21–2).
- *Shorter-term focus* The new system was based on agreed 'Survey' and Treasury figures for a nine-year spread: five past years, the current year and three future years. In the Survey, past expenditure had to be justified and 'there were no absolutely inescapable commitments' (Thain and Wright 1995: 260). Departments could then bid for additional resources for the next 3 years (1995: 261). In reality the important 'bids' were for next year's spending, and therefore the system was in some ways a return to the pre-PESC annual process (1995: 289)
- *Complete shift to cash planning.* In 1982 volume planning was abandoned. This was meant to provide ministers with an incentive to use their cash allocation in the most efficient manner possible, especially when the MTFS underestimated inflation, and cash limits had a built-in 'efficiency' gain of 0.5 per cent (Thain and Wright 1995: 254 and 259).
- *Increased emphasis on value-for-money* Thatcher appointed a businessman, Sir Derek Rayner, to advise her on efficiency and to lead an efficiency strategy unit located in her Office. This strategy effectively replaced the discredited PAR system, producing one-off efficiency scrutinies designed to reduce the cost of delivering the output of programmes (Thain and Wright 1995: 254 and 259).

The development of the public expenditure system under the Conservatives reflected their ideological concerns: to reduce the size and cost of the public sector and control inflation. The development of cash limits plus efficiency scrutinies was intended to provide ministers with incentives to use public monies efficiently and effectively.

In 1997 a new Labour Government again revamped the system to meet its own 'Third Way' priorities. It drew on elements of the previous system but used them to invest in and expand public services. The architects of the New Labour system claimed it would enhance the rationality of spending by focusing 'on long-term planning and outputs rather than short-term bargaining and inputs' (Her Majesty's Treasury 1998: 1).

New Labour and the Comprehensive Spending Review

In 1997 the Chancellor of the Exchequer, Gordon Brown, revamped the Treasury role in overall management of the economy – delegating some of the key elements, such as monetary policy to prevent inflation growing beyond agreed levels, to the Bank of England. Having retained the previous Conservative Government's spending plans in 1997, in 1998 he launched his own Comprehensive Spending Review, based on three-year projections of (and plans for) spending, combined with Public Service Agreements (PSAs) that specified the outputs that should be gained from this spending. (We highlight key elements of the 2000 health PSA in box 3.5.) These Reviews set 'firm and fixed three-year Departmental Expenditure Limits and, through Public Service Agreements (PSA), define the key improvements that the public can expect from these resources' (Her Majesty's Treasury 2009).

The Comprehensive Spending Review represented a new type of relationship between the Treasury and spending departments. In exchange for additional resources, Departments would not only specify the key policy outcomes they aimed to achieve but also identify and implement ways of achieving such outcomes more efficiently. The Prime Minister, Blair, in his Foreword to the 1998 Review, referred to the new spending as money for modernisation and indicated that 'In *health* there will be massive investment but in return the NHS is expected to deliver more responsive, higher quality care, more modern equipment and to cut waiting lists' (Blair 1998, italics in the original).

Box 3.5   Public Service Agreement for Health and Social Care in England in 2000 (Source: Her Majesty's Treasury 2000)

Aims   The PSA indicated that the aim of spending was 'To transform the health and social care system so that it produces faster, fairer services that deliver better health and tackle health inequalities'.

Objectives   The PSA included four main objectives and performance targets:
- improving health outcomes for everyone
- improving patient and carer experience of the NHS and Social Services
- effective delivery of appropriate care
- fair access.

Specification of objectives and targets   Each of these objectives was specified in more detail with specific targets. Thus, the objective of improving health outcomes for everyone was divided into two more detailed areas:
- Reduce substantially the mortality rates from major killers by 2010: from heart disease by at least 40% in people under 75; from cancer by at least 20% in people under 75; and from suicide and undetermined injury by at least 20%. Key to the delivery of this target will be implementing the National Service Frameworks for Coronary Heart Disease and Mental Health and the National Cancer Plan.
- Narrow the health gap between socio-economic groups and between the most deprived areas and the rest of the country, in childhood and throughout life. Specific national targets will be developed in consultation with external stakeholders and experts and published in 2001 in time to become fully operational by the beginning of 2002-03.

Efficiency and value for money   The PSA included a statement on the ways in which the effectiveness of the use of health-care resources would be judged:
- The cost of care commissioned from Trusts which perform well against indicators of fair access, quality and responsiveness, will become the benchmark for the NHS. All will be expected to reach the level of the best over the next five years, with agreed milestones for 2003–4.

An important aspect of the new system was a commitment
to continual review and reform to generate sustained improvement in the outputs of public services. These reviews built on
innovation in public-sector management, such as New Public
Management that involved the creation of explicit standards and
measurement of performance alongside an emphasis on the control
of outputs (Osborne and McLaughlin 2000: 9). Such measure-
ments provided a way of comparing quantified input (money)
with quantified output (services or benefit to the public), thereby
reviewing the effectiveness of past decisions. In addition to ad
hoc reviews and zero-based budgeting exercises (Her Majesty's
Treasury 2006: 4), the Treasury regularly monitored the performance of departments against their PSA targets: 'The Government
monitors progress against PSA targets, and departments report in
detail twice a year in their annual Departmental Reports (published
in spring) and in their autumn performance reports' (Her Majesty's
Treasury n.d.).

Periodic Comprehensive Spending Reviews covering three-year
periods have become an established part of spending allocation and
control, with reviews in 1998, 2000, 2002, 2004 and 2007 (Her
Majesty's Treasury 2009). A further review was due in either 2009
or 2010 but it was delayed until after the general election of May
2010. This delay indicated that the outgoing Labour Government
was reluctant to publish information indicating the extent of the cuts
in public expenditure that would be necessary to deal with the consequences of the 'credit crunch' in 2007 and the impact of bailing out
the banks and the subsequent recession on public finances.

Spending on health In 1997 Gordon Brown restricted spending on health care to the levels set by the previous Conservative
Government. As the Prime Minister noted in 1998, 'we have stuck
rigidly to tough spending plans since the Election' (Blair 1998). To
avoid conflict over this decision, the Prime Minister appointed Frank
Dobson as Secretary of State for Health, who was seen as someone
who would accept short-term restrictions on spending. Despite this
early restraint, health was the most favoured programme (1997–
2010) and health expenditure increased substantially in each of the
spending reviews.

The 2007 Spending Review announced further substantial
increases in NHS spending. As box 3.6 indicates, these were
justified in terms of improved quality and quantity of services provided and the promise of future improvements in efficiency and
effectiveness.

Box 3.6　Summary of the key elements of the 2007 Comprehensive Spending Review – proposed service improvement for the health and social care expenditure (Source: Her Majesty's Treasury 2007)

Increase in spending　The 2007 Comprehensive Spending Review planned to increase NHS spending by 4 per cent per year, taking the budget from £90 billion in 2007–8 to £110 billion by 2010–11. There were also planned 'efficiency savings' of at least £8.2 billion.

Purpose of the spending　To create an NHS that was fair, personalised, effective, safe and locally accountable.

Targets　These included:
- improved access to GP services, with additional resources for over 100 new GP practices in the 25 per cent of Primary Care Trusts (PCTs) with the poorest provision, and 150 new health centres open seven days a week;
- cleaner hospitals, with the introduction of MRSA screening for all elective patients next year, and for all emergency admissions as soon as practicable within the next three years, deep cleaning of hospitals and increased powers for matrons and ward sisters to report concerns; and
- a more innovative NHS, with a new Health Innovation Council to drive innovation, increasing Research and Development spending to over £1 billion by 2010–11.

Given the limitations of earlier systems of allocating public expenditure, did the system of Comprehensive Spending Reviews achieve the holy grail of fully rational spending decisions? At the level of rhetoric, it certainly appears as though this is the case. For the first time there is a clear articulation of the objectives which spending is expected to achieve (Public Service Agreements). The movement to periodic Comprehensive Spending Reviews signalled the end of annual bargaining, allowing more time and energy to be devoted to predicting and planning spending. At the same time the various reviews and zero-based budgeting exercises have provided opportunities to review past decisions and historic expenditure. However, the system fell short of full rationality. As we noted, there has been a continuing increase in health spending but this continued spending was based on a political judgement that health spending was more popular than (for example) defence spending. It was not grounded in a comparison of the relative benefits of heath versus defence spending, which is impossible.

For ten years, the Labour Government 'oversaw' steady economic growth which created resources and allowed for regular reviews that demonstrated increased spending and the benefits it would generate for the UK population. This was particularly evident in the reviews that took place in the run-up to general elections (2000 and 2004). However, in autumn 2007 the Government's luck ran out as the 'credit crunch' signalled the start of an economic recession. In such circumstances the Government became more reticent about spending, replacing the public announcements of increased spending with covert bilateral negotiations between the Chief Secretary and spending Ministers over cuts in expenditure.

The Coalition Government: was it rational to protect health spending?

In May 2010, following an indecisive general election, the Conservative and Liberal Democrats formed a Coalition Government. The two parties agreed that the existing level of public expenditure was unsustainable and that over the five-year period of the Parliament, the deficit should be substantially reduced, with immediate cuts of £6 billion in the financial year 2010/11. The parties agreed that spending on the NHS would increase in each year of the Parliament as would the target of spending 0.7 per cent of Gross National Income on overseas aid. They agreed there would be an emergency budget within 50 days of the signing of the Coalition agreement, and full spending review would be completed by the autumn (Liberal Democrats 2010).

During the summer of 2010 all spending ministers and their civil servants, apart from those responsible for the health and overseas aid budgets, were invited to discuss with the Treasury Ministers and civil servants how they planned to reduce their budgets by 25 per cent over a five-year period (Curtis 2010).

The results of these negotiations formed the basis of the Spending Review which the Chancellor of the Exchequer presented to Parliament and published in October 2010 (Her Majesty's Treasury 2010). The Review stated that all departmental budgets apart from health and overseas aid were being cut by an average of 19 per cent, or £81 billion of planned expenditure, over the remaining four years of the Parliament. This would enable the Government to eliminate the structural budget deficit within five years. The cuts were actually calculated using planned expenditure with the expenditure of 2010/11 as a baseline. Thus, if current plans and policies agreed in 2010/11 and costing £698.8 billion per annum had been continued until 2014/15, the forecast expenditure would have been £739.8 billion per annum. The Spending Review had set an overall limit or envelope of £660.9 billion, an overall reduction of 8 per cent (Her Majesty's Treasury 2010: 17). In the settlement the budgets of health and overseas aid were protected. It was agreed that the health budget would increase from £103.8 billion in 2010/11 to £114.4 in 2014/15, and this would include an additional £1 billion to support social care through the health budget (Her Majesty's Treasury 2010: 43). In contrast, planned expenditure for other departments was substantially reduced, and they had to make major policy changes to reduce planned expenditure. For example, the budget for the Department of Business, Innovation and Skills was cut from £18.6 billion in 2010/11 to £14.6 billion in 2014/15. One of the major policy changes which the Department made was in higher education 'to shift a greater proportion of funding from the taxpayer to the individuals who benefit' (Her Majesty's Treasury 2010: 51), by allowing universities in England to raise student tuition fees from £3,000 to £9,000 a year.

In some respects the 2010 Review can be considered to be instrumentally rational. The Coalition had agreed that the public expenditure deficit would be substantially reduced, and as long as there are no unanticipated economic or political developments then the Review should enable the Coalition to achieve its objective. However, in doing this the Coalition reversed the normal relationship between money and social policy. Money is normally a means of achieving policy ends. However, in the context of the 2010 Review, policy changes such as the increase in university tuition fees were a means of achieving financial ends, the deficit reduction. The protection of the health budget was important in political terms for the Coalition, and particularly the Conservative Party. However, in rational terms it was difficult to justify. Protecting the health and overseas aid budget meant that, to achieve an average reduction of 8 per cent, some departments had to reduce their planned expenditure by well over 20 per cent, distorting spending choices (O'Grady 2011: 32). Such uneven cuts were unlikely to have minimised the overall

reduction of benefits to the citizens of the UK. Before the 2011
election, Vince Cable, a senior Liberal Democrat politician publicly
criticised the Conservative Party proposals to protect NHS spending,
arguing they risked protecting inefficient spending in health while
imposing cuts on other relatively efficient and beneficial spending
programmes (O'Grady 2011: 32). After the election, as Secretary of
State for Business, Innovation and Skills, he was a major 'loser' in the
spending review.

Comment

In principle, money provides the basis for rational policy making.
It enables the comparison of the inputs and outputs of different programmes and for making decisions based on the most
beneficial allocations. In reality the complexity and uncertainties
of policies and price changes mean that fully rational zero-based
budgeting, in which all previous decisions are reviewed, is very
much an aspiration. Rationality only exists at the margins, in decisions over increments of increased spending or specific cuts in
spending.

KEY POINTS

- The key decision makers in spending allocations aspire to
  rationality and the architects of each new system of allocation
  claim it will distribute funds more rationally than the previous
  system.
- Given the difficulties of predicting the future (for example,
  ministers and civil servants planning spending in 2007 had no
  knowledge of the credit crunch and its impact) and the complexity of decision making, it is difficult to create a rational system of
  allocation.
- The system for allocating public spending in the UK has been
  restructured several times since the Second World War. There has
  been clear evidence of learning: the PESC system was designed to
  overcome the limitations and stop–go effects of annual spending
  decisions; when PESC exacerbated the financial difficulties of the
  1970s then a cash limits system provided a more focused approach
  to spending decisions.
- Although ministers and civil servants aspire to rationality, in spending considerations such as the 2010 Spending Review, rationality is

severely bounded by political judgements and negotiations and is
evident only at the margins of decisions.

4

Power and influence in policy making: policy communities and networks

AIMS

To examine the ways in which health policy makers can overcome limitations in expertise by broadening participation in policy making, and the influence this has on the nature of rationality.

OBJECTIVES

- To consider the nature of knowledge in policy making, and various models for enhancing expertise and knowledge and the impact which these can have on the rationality of policy making
- To examine the ways in which health policy makers build and support policy communities and networks to facilitate access to expertise and broaden participation in policy making
- To consider the ways in which participation in health policy making has changed over time and the impact of these changes on policy making.

Rationality in policy making requires knowledge both of the purposes that policy is designed to achieve and of the most effective means of achieving these ends. In chapter 2 we noted that in UK government there is a knowledge deficit. Ministers who are formally responsible for policy making are not expected to have in-depth knowledge of the policy areas they are responsible for. They are supported by civil servants and special advisers who can help them overcome this knowledge deficit. However, even this range of expertise is restricted – for example, while policy advisers located in

Whitehall may have extensive general knowledge of health they are
likely to lack in-depth knowledge of specific issues or localities. Thus
policy makers need to be able to access more specialised knowledge and this may involve the development of policy networks and
communities.

4.1 Rationality, knowledge and expertise

Policy networks and communities: accessing knowledge

In principle, the more knowledge that policy makers can access, the
greater the rationality of policies. However, as we noted in chapter
3, accessing knowledge can be a costly and time-consuming process
and therefore policy makers need to be able to access appropriate
knowledge as quickly and as cheaply as possible. One way of doing
this is through networks of individuals and groups who are willing
to provide advice, usually at minimal or no cost. As Kingdom notes,
groups with a special interest in an issue are likely to 'be first with
expertise and information' when a new problem develops, that when
'AIDS began its fateful march through the population, the Terrence
Higgins Foundation clearly understood the problem better than the
mandarins' (1999: 511).

Relatively stable and on-going relations between civil servants
and individuals and groups with an expertise and interest in specific policy issues tend to develop around particular policy areas,
sectors and issues (Rhodes 1997: 29). The membership and nature
of the network varies from context to context: 'A policy network can
include ministers, civil servants, special advisers . . . , pressure group
representatives, etc. Around each policy – be it health, defence,
welfare policy for lone parents, asylum seekers etc. – a different
network will exist with a different range of actors involved' (Richards
and Smith 2002: 21).

While each policy issue has its own unique network, since issues
are not independent, over time these networks (especially their inner
circle) can develop into established and stable policy communities
– i.e. experts inside and outside government who interact regularly
over different but related issues. Thus, those involved in policy networks have different levels of participation, with the core of ministers
and their advisers having a full-time engagement in and accountability for policy making. They are regularly consulted as policy makers
anticipate this will yield high benefits (access to knowledge) and
low cost and risk (they trust insiders not to leak information about

emerging policies). While they also consult outsiders, it is likely to be on an ad hoc basis – when they require specific information – and they are likely to consult them later in the policy-making process. Outsiders are not trusted to abide by the implicit rules of the game, such as confidentiality, and therefore may leak sensitive information to the media if they think this will assist their interests. Thus insider and outsider groups can be differentiated not only in their usefulness but also in their perceived legitimacy. Insider groups, through their on-going relations with the inner core of policy makers, not only have proved their usefulness but also are perceived as legitimate in that they share the norms, values, interests and culture of core policy makers. Kingdom mapped six major policy networks in the UK. His inner core of health policy makers included the Prime Minister, health ministers and their advisers. The insider groups who were regularly consulted included health authorities such as Strategic Health Authorities, important suppliers of the NHS such as drug companies and representatives of major professional groups such as the medical Royal Colleges and the British Medical Association. The outsider groups who were only consulted occasionally and on special issues included associations representing alternative practitioners and groups representing patients and health-care consumers (Kingdom 1991: 421).

Policy networks and particularly communities can be seen as an important component of a rational policy-making system. They enable key policy makers such as ministers and civil servants to rapidly access a range of expertise. They are informal and low-cost, and can operate swiftly. They have stability and continuity. They are a way of accessing collective, accumulated knowledge and therefore of learning from past errors and experiences. They can help reduce the barrier between policy formation and implementation – e.g., if the BMA is involved in policy making it can gain the support of its members, particularly general practitioners, in its implementation.

The view that the more knowledge policy makers have, the more rational policy making becomes, is based on a positivistic approach to knowledge. In this positivist framework scientific methods enable the collection of facts that provide an objective picture or understanding of reality, so the more facts the better. In this perspective it does not really matter who collects the facts or makes the policies as long as they use the right methods. Thus, as we noted in our initial discussion of rational methods of policy making, the emphasis is on the process rather than particular participants in the process. If you look at Jenkins's diagrammatic representation of a rational policy-making system (figure 2.1 in chapter 2) or DEFRA's diagram representing the ways evidence should be used in policy making (figure 2.3 in chapter 2) you will see that they describe elements of process such as reviewing knowledge or evidence, but the actual policy makers are invisible.

However, even using the scientific method does not guarantee 'objectivity'. Using scientific methods, individuals and groups can create very different versions of reality. As we note in chapter 5 (see box 5.1), in the early 1990s the scientific consensus was that 'mad cow disease' did not pose a threat to human health, though some 'maverick' scientists did not agree and subsequent events showed that the consensus was wrong. In the case of the Measles, Mumps and Rubella (MMR) vaccine, in 1998 Andrew Wakefield and his colleagues at a London teaching hospital published an article in the *Lancet* based on 'scientific evidence' of a link between the MMR vaccine and childhood autism. Although this article was subsequently retracted, anti-vaccine campaign groups such as Jabs maintain the link exists (Alaszewski 2011).

If there is no single version of reality but alternative and competing ones, then these differences cannot be resolved by more knowledge, but have to be resolved politically through the exercise of power, with one version becoming the dominant version and the one which provides the framework for policy making. In the next section we will explore the ways in which the knowledge accessed and promoted by insider and outsider groups differs and consider the ways in which power is exercised.

Policy communities versus policy networks: knowledge, power and rationality

The difference between insider and outsider groups influences the nature and frequency of participation in policy making. This differentiation relates to two types of knowledge: abstract and personal knowledge (Lam 2000). Abstract knowledge is technical knowledge that is developed through scientific research or through professional practice; in the health area, epidemiology is an important source of abstract knowledge. Personal knowledge is concrete and grounded in individual face-to-face experience and finds expression in feelings and emotions such as trust and distrust. As we have already noted, the stability of relationships between core policy makers and insiders is based on a mixture of abstract knowledge, technical expertise and personal knowledge, particularly trust. While networks are likely to have a mix of different types of interactions, communications and relations, if relatively stable personal trust-based relations exist, then participants form a policy community which is collectively engaged in policy formation. However, if the network is relatively unstable with changing membership and evidence of distrust, such as overt conflict, then interaction is likely to be more restricted and relationships potentially involve conflict.

Rhodes (1997: 35–45) has argued that policy communities and issue networks are two ends of a continuum, but that these two extremes have identifiable features. Participation in policy communities is restricted and membership is relatively stable – indeed, certain 'difficult' groups are deliberately excluded – while participation in issue networks is open and membership fluctuates. Policy communities tend to be integrated, with members interacting frequently on policy matters and sharing values and accepting the legitimacy of the outcomes. Issue networks tend to be fragmented, with disagreement over values, and conflict and disputes over outcomes. In policy communities, resources and power tend to be balanced and the development of policy involves exchange and negotiations. In contrast, in the issue network the inner core tends to dominate resources and the network and to make key decisions, so interactions take the form of consultation rather than negotiation. Outsiders tend not to share the same background and therefore cannot be expect to understand and abide by the rules of the game. Thus in the early stages of the AIDS epidemic, representatives of the Terrence Higgins Trust were mainly younger gay men from a variety of social backgrounds who did not observe the conventions of the core groups, e.g. in dress or speech. Their otherness and potential dangerousness meant that they were treated with care and caution, especially in terms of the information that they were given, in case they made it available to the media.

The policy community fits well into the rational policy-making model. It provides access to expert knowledge while minimising both cost and conflict. This approach is restrictive, it limits participation to insiders and therefore, as we will note below and in chapter 7, is difficult to reconcile with the broader participation expected of a democratic society. A policy community can be seen as elitist as policy is formulated behind closed doors and participants are expected to understand and obey the rules of the policy game – especially that any information gained through participation in policy discussions is confidential and must not be made public. Generally such rules are unwritten and unstated.

This system is rational as long as those inside the group are seen as having a monopoly on relevant knowledge and those excluded do not have important knowledge which could and should be part of the process of policy making. Major failures of policy tend to indicate that policy communities, especially those narrowly grounded in scientific knowledge, have missed important information. We note in chapter 5 that, in the BSE/vCJD disaster (see box 5.1), the Department of Health relied heavily on expert advice and, failing to recognise that such advice was both limited and flawed, tended to select those advisers and that advice which suited its purpose of reassuring the public about the safety of agriculture and beef production in the UK:

> The report of the Inquiry into that animal and human tragedy [the BSE disaster] paints a graphic picture of a particularly diseased form of club government, in which those responsible for food safety were bound together with powerful economic interests in a closed collusive world . . . Food safety control is an area historically dominated by powerful corporate actors with key allies in the state machine. (Moran 2003: 149).

In the case of the pesticide DDT, scientific and commercial interests established a consensus that the chemical was safe. Concerned US citizens such as Rachel Carson collected evidence to show that DDT was harmful to the environment, stimulating a presidential investigation and a major policy change, and providing a focus for the emerging ecology movement (see box 4.1).

The barriers which policy communities create to alternative outsider perspectives undermine the rationality of policy making. This exercise of power maintains a dominant perspective. Insiders tend to see the world in the same way, and challenges to this worldview, especially from outsider groups, are thwarted. Thus policy making is a political process in which the stability and the status quo are maintained in the face of destabilising pressure from outsider groups. Moran argues that, until the 'great policy crisis' (2003: 4) of the 1970s, policy communities – or in his terms a 'club system' – dominated policy making in the UK. This system was 'oligarchic, informal and secretive' (2003: 4) and pervaded all areas of policy making and implementation.

As policy communities restrict participation to a trusted inner

Box 4.1   DDT, Rachel Carson, *Silent Spring* and the development of the ecology movement

Historical context   DDT (dichlorodiphenyltrichloroethane) is a chemical synthesised in 1874 and found in 1939 to be an effective pesticide that could kill mosquitoes and lice and so reduce the incidence of malaria and typhus, and functions as an insecticide in agriculture. DDT was used during the 1940s to help war efforts in Europe and the South Pacific, and in 1955 the World Health Organization started a campaign to eliminate malaria. The scientific consensus was that DDT was a safe and effective chemical and the policy communities in both health and agriculture endorsed its widespread use.

Public concern and alternative evidence   In the 1950s there were concerns about the widespread spraying of DDT. In 1957, residents of Long Island New York went to court to try to prevent the US Department of Agriculture spraying DDT, and in 1958 a resident of Massachusetts wrote to the *Boston Herald* indicating that DDT spraying was killing birds on her property. Rachel Carson, who had been concerned about spraying in the Pacific in the 1940s, had been gathering evidence on the harmful effects of DDT and reacted by publishing *Silent Spring* (Carson 1962). This was a critique of both DDT, which created reproductive problems for birds, and the chemical policy community in which the claims of industry scientists were uncritically accepted by government officials.

Change in policy and policy making   *Silent Spring* had an immediate and major impact, attracting the attention of the media and politicians. President Kennedy instructed his scientific committee to investigate and they confirmed most of Carson's concerns about DDT. The campaign to ban DDT became a major focus for the developing environmental movement, which used the courts in the USA to exert pressure on regulators. DDT was banned in the USA in 1972 and in the UK in 1982.

circle, they exclude potentially valuable expertise and knowledge. Broadening participation may not only improve rationality in terms of better access to knowledge but it can also improve rationality in terms of the greater acceptability of policy. As Ham and Hill (1993:

85) have argued, the test of a good policy is not whether it is rational for the policy maker and achieves his or her objectives but whether it is acceptable and 'whether the policy secures the agreement of the interests involved'.

Thus networks provide the basis for broader participation and pluralism rather than elitism in policy making. Advocates of such pluralism argue that core policy makers should consult widely so that both expertise and its underpinning assumptions and values are fully exposed. This builds on Lindblom's insight that policy making cannot be reduced to a technical or economic activity but forms part of broader social and political processes: 'formal processes of analysis and theory-building – no matter how desirable – are inevitably mediated by processes of political interaction, and *are no substitute for them*' (Gregory 1993: 212–13 and 229, italics added).

Thus in the pluralistic framework the optimum policy is not necessarily the one that experts believe will achieve the best outcomes, but the one which commands the most support from competing interests. If all interests are represented, and if they have articulated their interests effectively, then this should also produce the best outcomes (Habermas 1987). Pluralism emphasises the political interaction between competing groups. As Kingdom states, in pluralism, policy making is a political process as 'Public policy is the outcome, or resultant, of a number of group forces acting against each other. This may be compared with a mathematical vector diagram in which the *resultant* reflects the combination effect of all other forces . . . Thus the system tends towards a state of equilibrium, with all forces having some effect on the outcome' (1991: 418).

Ministers and civil servants can play two different roles in the pluralist system. In one version of pluralism they are participants, representing their own interests and contributing to the policy debate. In the other they stand outside the policy arena and ensure that all interests are represented (with none getting an unfair advantage) and help to locate the policy solution that provides the maximum satisfaction to all interests (Kingdom 1991: 419). The pluralist model acknowledges that knowledge is spread between different groups and not monopolised by an elite and that policy making is not just a technical exercise in processing knowledge but involves interaction and negotiation. The differences between the two models are outlined in table 4.1.

Table 4.1   Elitism versus pluralism

	Elitism	Pluralism
Process	Closed, access restricted	Open, publicly accessible
Participation	Insider groups	Multiple groups
Scope of participation	Only dominant interests represented	All interests articulated
Role of policy core	Key players	'Referee'
Perception of knowledge	Key knowledge held by experts	Knowledge diffused between groups

Elitism or pluralism: the corporatist approach to government and policy making

The discussion of policy communities and issue networks in the last section focused on the processes and groups in particular policy areas such as health. However interaction between such groups can be expanded into negotiations and bargaining over a broader range of issues. In the corporatist approach, the government seeks to identify and bargain with groups representing major sections of the population and 'elected politicians make public policy with the key organised interests in society (usually big business and organised labour), who then share responsibility for implementing the agreed policies' (Dearlove and Saunders 2000: 763–4).

This approach to government's role in policy making was used in fascist states, such as Italy in the 1920s and 1930s, where the state created and used corporations to by-pass democratic institutions such as political parties. After the Second World War, democratic states such as Sweden and Austria used this approach to develop social democratic welfare states. The United Kingdom in the 1960s and 1970s experimented with this approach as a way of dealing with social and economic problems, for example restraining wage increases and associated inflation that were a by-product of the Keynesian demand management and full employment (see chapter 3 and Dearlove and Saunders 2000: 512–24). This approach culminated in the 'Social Contract' when Prime Minister Jim Callaghan responded to the economic and policy crisis of the late 1970s by negotiating an agreement with the trade unions and employers' associations to control prices and wages, in exchange for increased public spending and benefits. The agreement collapsed in the 'Winter of Discontent' of 1978/9, and the election of a Conservative

Government led by Margaret Thatcher ended the corporatist experiment.

Corporatism can be seen as a modified form of elitism. The government does recognise and negotiate with some groups but only the most powerful ones, especially those that can veto government policy and prevent its implementation (see chapter 6 for a discussion of veto power). Thus, for key policy makers, corporatism is a way of simplifying the policy-making process: excluding the wide range of groups which do not have power and negotiating behind closed doors with the key groups who can really influence the outcome (Dearlove and Saunders 2000: 522).

Cawson (1986) and Saunders (1984) have argued that pluralism and corporatism co-exist in the UK but operate at different levels of policy making and perform different functions. They argued that at central national level, where key investment decisions are made about the allocation of resources between and within policy areas, corporatism is a good description of the ways in which the elite make decisions behind closed doors. Consumption decisions that relate to ways in which such resources are distributed between competing groups of beneficiaries involve more groups in a more open, localised format and thus are more pluralistic. Thus they saw policy making as having an inner corporatist core with an outer pluralistic periphery (see Cawson 1986). Cawson's and Saunders's differentiation between investment and consumption policy reflects Walt's (1994) differentiation between high politics (major issues that attract government attention because an error can threaten the government) and low politics (routine administrative issues that can be dealt with locally), though Walt's duality does not specifically relate to investment versus consumption decisions.

Key policy makers can be seen as reluctant collaborators in policy communities. They collaborate and negotiate with groups outside the inner policy core because they have to. They need the resources that these groups possess. The main resource is knowledge but, as we will note in chapter 6, some groups have veto power to block the implementation of policy and others can endorse and therefore increase the legitimacy of policies.

A policy community can be seen as an extension of the inner policy core. Insiders are co-opted into the policy-making system. They can influence decisions at an early formative stage but have to accept the rule of the game – i.e. secretive decision making – and to an extent are committed to the policy which they have helped create. In contrast, outsider groups who cannot be trusted are perceived as lacking useful resources, they are seen as different to those in the inner policy core and excluded.

Issue networks, on the other hand, are based on a more positive commitment to and recognition of the intrinsic value of participation. Not only do key policy makers accept they do not have a monopoly on key resources but they also accept that it is difficult to identify all necessary resources. Thus, in terms of knowledge, while it is possible to identify some deficits or gaps, there are also deficits that are difficult to identify, i.e. the 'unknown unknowns'. Thus, the process of collaboration can have unexpected benefits but can also improve policy by increasing agreement and support for policies.

4.2 Participation in health policy making: from elitism to a more open system

Participation in the 1940s and 1950s: the era of the club culture

When the NHS was established in the 1940s, government accepted responsibility for the funding of health care but accepted that most of health policy related to highly technical activities which required the input of expertise from the medical profession. Nye Bevan, the radical reforming Labour minister, established the overall approach of engaging key medical groups in the health policy process. There were on-going and confidential discussions with the BMA which had started as soon as it became evident in 1943 that the state was going to take on major responsibility for health care (Eckstein 1960: 74). However, when the BMA effectively withdrew its cooperation, Bevan negotiated the final structure of the service with the elite of the profession: the presidents of the Royal Colleges (see box 4.2, and we discuss the nature of the Royal Colleges and their veto power in chapter 6).

Eckstein (1960: 24–5) noted that Bevan was responding to the dominant policy-making culture, of which there were three key aspects:

- *Underlying corporatism* based on views that: society is made up of distinctive groups with common interests and occupational or other identities; and policies should be informed by conversations with representatives of the corporations/sectors likely to be affected by them;
- *Deference to the technical expertise of professionals* Key policy makers, Ministers and civil servants accepted that doctors possessed skills

---

Box 4.2　Nye Bevan and the formation of the NHS

Context　Following the 1942 Beveridge Report and the election victory in 1945, the Labour Government was committed to the creation of a National Health Service.

Participants　These included the Minister, Nye Bevan, his civil servants and representatives of the medical profession – especially the Presidents of the Royal Colleges. In the final discussions the BMA was marginalised as it was articulating GP hostility to the new service and their anxieties about becoming 'salaried' state employees.

Process　Bevan required both the cooperation and expertise of the Royal Colleges especially for the crucial part of the policy – nationalising hospitals – but also to overcome resistance from General Practitioners who were threatening to boycott the new service.

Policy outcomes　Bevan accepted the Royal Colleges' advice that the hospital service should be modelled on the voluntary hospitals, with a teaching hospital at the core of each region and other hospitals grouped together, and all hospital medical staff forming part of a Consultant's team. He accepted advice that GPs should enter the service as independent contractors, with contracts to provide general medical services for patients on their lists, not as salaried employees.

---

and knowledge of policy and practice which they did not have and which they needed;

- *Delegation of authority* to key individuals in both government and professional bodies to represent, communicate and negotiate as they saw fit. Thus civil servants, in most circumstances, could act on behalf of ministers, and talking to the BMA was treated as equivalent to talking to all doctors.

There were also several health-specific factors which reinforced the deference of policy makers to the medical profession:

- *Weakness of the Ministry of Health within government* Paradoxically the formation of the NHS weakened the Ministry. In the 1920s and 1930s it had been a multi-purpose Ministry that played a lead role in state health and welfare provision. Following the formation of the NHS its remit was restricted and, given the continued challenges of funding the NHS, its dependency on the Treasury increased. It was 'a relatively minor department' (Eckstein 1960: 54).

• *The predominant position of the medical profession amongst the professional groups providing health care* Although the medical profession was internally divided, especially between general practitioners who were represented by the BMA, and hospital specialists – who were also represented by the BMA but had their own separate Royal Colleges – the profession had established a pre-eminent position within the health-care system. While other occupational groups such as nurses had substantially more members, none were as well organised and effectively represented, or had the veto power of the doctors.

The formation of the NHS and other parts of the welfare state in the 1940s stimulated the activities of groups which stood to gain from policy, in terms either of income or of benefits. Eckstein noted that 'if interaction among politically active groups produces policy, policy in turn creates politically active groups' (1960: 27), and in the 1940s the medical profession used the opportunity provided by the formation of the NHS to develop a close relationship with both central policy makers and local administrators. Eckstein described the way in which the new service provided opportunities through professional partcipation in advisory bodies at national and local level. At the local level, the Local Medical Committees, which Executive Councils had to consult over the administration of general practitioner services, were effectively local committees of the BMA (Eckstein 1960: 46).

At national level, the Ministry of Health and the BMA developed a close informal working partnership. In some ways the structures of the two organisations were aligned, with members of the BMA hierarchies linked to their equivalents or 'alter egos' within the Ministry of Health (Eckstein 1960: 84–5). The BMA representatives developed close relationships with their counterparts. Eckstein (1960: 89) noted that they sometimes referred to their Ministry counterparts as 'our colleagues' and were on intimate first-name terms. While relationships between counterparts could be tense with 'charges and counter-charges' – especially when the issues under discussion related to the most sensitive policy issues, doctors' pay and conditions (Eckstein 1960: 88–9) – typical relations were relaxed and club-like: 'Most negotiations . . . are "intimate" not only in that they are friendly but also they are highly private – out of the public limelight and insulated against both interdepartmental relations and pressure from the grass roots of the profession' (Eckstein 1960: 88).

The most important issues tended to be discussed with the greatest informality, as formal procedures would 'inhibit bargaining and the free exchange of views' (Eckstein 1960: 86). These intimate, informal and on-going relations were 'backstairs networks' (Eckstein 1960: 89). Through such networks, the medical profession was closely involved not only in the detailed development of health policy but also in the administration of the NHS. It was accordingly 'a vital part of the departmental decision-making machinery' (Eckstein 1960: 78). Thus Ministers of Health effectively gave the BMA a veto in all areas of health policy and the BMA was informed of, and negotiated over, virtually every decision.

There were episodes of conflict that the media and public became aware of. These generally took place when key participants needed to involve others in the decision making. Relatively rarely – often over doctors' terms and conditions – civil servants needed to involve ministers and the Treasury, and the BMA needed to consult their membership (Eckstein 1960: 88) (in chapter 1 we discussed the early conflict between GPs and the Ministry that went public and had to be resolved by outside arbitration: see box 1.5). In contrast, even fairly complex issues that involved detailed bargaining could be successfully resolved through the use of negotiations when the backstairs network reinforced more public discussions. In box 4.3 we discuss the BMA's successful negotiation over redundant Registrars.

In the 1940s and 1950s the formation of health policy involved an elitist partnership between the Ministry of Health and the medical profession, particularly the BMA. The relationship between the medical profession and the Ministry was similar to that described by Selznick (1949) in his study of a US New Deal programme in the Tennessee Valley. The programme involved the construction of a major dam to produce electricity and help poor rural farmers. To overcome local opposition, important local landowners were co-opted into the administration of the programme, allowing them to shape it to their interests. In the early period of the NHS, the medical profession was also co-opted and was similarly able to shape policies to suit its interests. Thus, health policy making was enmeshed in a professional network which, as Rhodes (1997: 38) has noted, was highly stable, had restricted membership and served the interests of the profession.

**Box 4.3   The case of the redundant Registrars 1950–1958
(Eckstein 1960: 113–25)**

Historical context   When the NHS was established in 1948, Bevan accepted the recommendations of the Royal Colleges that the medical staffing structure of all the hospitals should follow the pattern established in the elite voluntary hospitals, where senior, experienced specialists were appointed to Consultant posts and all other doctors held time-limited posts (Registrar or House Officer) as trainees. The practical problems of creating the service meant that some older doctors who were not seen as suitable for Consultant appointments were given Registrar posts. The failure to expand specialist appointments meant that younger doctors were not able to progress through the training grades to Consultant appointments. These career blockages meant that the Ministry was funding unnecessary posts.

Initial Ministry proposal   In 1950 the Ministry produced a proposal to remedy the problem of career blockage. It estimated that in the foreseeable future there would be 1,700 new Consultant appointments (approximately 150 a year) and therefore there should be 1,700 Registrars in training. This meant that 1,100 Registrars were surplus to requirements and should be made redundant. The Ministry discussed these proposals with representatives of the Joint Committee for Specialists (JSC) (a BMA / Royal Colleges Committee) which apparently accepted them, and the policy was issued as a memorandum to Regional Hospital Boards.

Pressure from the medical profession   The medical profession reacted critically and publicly to the proposal and sympathetic MPs raised the issue in the House of Commons. In the adjournment debate in December 1950, Bevan defended the proposal, arguing that the number of doctors in junior and training posts had to be aligned to future demand for Consultants, but he also suspended the memorandum, thus opening the way for negotiations. These were initiated by the Registrar's committee of the JSC in January 1951 and there followed extensive formal and backstairs negotiations lasting into 1954.

The final compromise   The Ministry stood by the principle that all junior doctors should be trainees on fixed-term contracts but allowed Regional Hospital Boards to extend the contracts of redundant Registrars in some cases until 1959. The number of redundancies was reduced and the number of posts was frozen at 1955 levels. Despite this, the relationship between training and Consultant posts remained unbalanced.

Dismantling the club culture in the 1970s and 1980s

The 1970s and 1980s were periods of economic turbulence with major recessions in 1973–6 and 1979–83. Political conflict marked the break-up of the post-war political consensus and was linked to major changes in policy-making culture and practices. Key features of these changes included:

- *Movement away from corporatism to political liberalism* The failure of the 'Social Contract' in the 1978/9 'Winter of Discontent' signalled a major shift in political culture. The incoming Conservative Government led by Margaret Thatcher was hostile to the trade unions that were partners in corporatist negotiations, and emphasised that the key relationship in a liberal democracy should be between Government and individual citizens.
- *Decline of deference to professionals* The special status of professionals as neutral objective experts was subject to scrutiny, with economists arguing that in many areas of production they formed cartels – restricting competition and maintaining artificially high prices.
- *Centralisation of authority* The culture of the civil service was subject to criticism and was increasingly seen by politicians as a cause of the long-term economic decline of the UK. Radical Ministers tended to see the civil service as a barrier to change. These views resulted in both increased political control – Mrs Thatcher expected her ministers to make key decisions – and more focused policy making (in chapter 2, we discussed the development of departmental boards to provide policy 'leadership').

There were also major changes that undermined the privileged position which the medical profession had enjoyed in policy making:

- *Strengthening of the position of the Department of Health within government* In the 1960s the position of the Ministry changed from that of a relatively minor Ministry to that of a major player and the lead Ministry in social welfare. This partially reflected a shift in attitudes to welfare at the end of the 1950s, with investment in and expansion of welfare through programmes such as hospital building, but it also reflected the restructuring of government at the end of the 1960s with the formation of superministries departments, such as the Department of Health and Social Security, to provide better coordination of policy.

- *Challenges to the dominant position of the medical profession in the delivery of health care* In the 1970s the organisation of other occupational groups in the health-care field improved substantially. Some occupations enhanced their standing through a professionalisation strategy, others through unionisation – e.g. ancillary workers (see below for the role of unions in the 1974 pay bed dispute) – and others, such as nurses, combined professionalisation with unionisation (as we note in chapter 5, several of the hospital scandals of the 1970s and 1980s started with industrial action by nurses). At the same time the role and status of 'administrators' in local health services increased as they became health services managers, enabling them to challenge the monopoly which doctors exercised over decision making. In a case study of a large hospital group in New York, Alford (1975) identified a similar process in which doctors formed a dominant elite and maintained the status quo, with policy making tending to favour their interests. Managers could challenge this dominance, especially when resources were restricted, as they were in the UK in the late 1970s and 1980s.
- *The development of the consumer movement* Alford (1975) also identified a third set of interests, those of consumers, but noted that these interests were repressed and marginalised and, when patients did organise, they were outsider groups that had to mobilise public support to exert any influence over policy. In the UK, such groups started to exert increasing influence, both locally and nationally.

The Labour Government of the late 1970s used corporatism as a response to economic crisis. In the health service this meant that the medical profession was no longer the sole or dominant partner in policy making. In some areas of policy, ministers and civil servants looked for other sources of expertise. For example, there was an increasing awareness in the late 1960s that, despite twenty years of state funding, resources were not evenly distributed between health regions in England. Richard Crossman first addressed the issue when he was Secretary of State, inviting Brian Abel-Smith as his special adviser to develop a formula for allocating resources equitably. In 1974 David Owen, the Labour Minister of Health, decided to refine the Crossman formula and created a working party which drew heavily on the expertise of NHS managers. The working party published its report (Department of Health and Social Security 1976b) and this became the basis of allocations in the NHS – representing a challenge to those medical practitioners working in the areas that had previously been well funded such as London.

In the Labour Government version of corporatism, participation was extended to groups that had often been excluded from policy making, especially the trade unions. In the area of health, this extension was evident in policy concerns such as the conflict over pay beds, a major issue during Barbara Castle's two-year period as Secretary of State for Social Services (1974–6). During the original negotiations with the medical profession over the NHS, Bevan conceded the right of hospital specialists to engage in private practice and to do so using NHS facilities, especially private or pay beds. In 1974 when a new teaching hospital, Charing Cross Hospital, was opened in West London, it included a dedicated wing for private patients. Following the restructuring of the service and tension over pay, the trade unions selected pay beds as an issue. In June 1974 the local National Union of Public Employees steward, Mrs Esther Brookstone – known in the media as the 'battling granny' – threatened strike action, and when in July the BMA threatened retaliation, local managers asked the Minister to intervene. Castle decided that pay beds represented unfinished business and indicated to the unions that, as soon as possible, the Government would pass legislation to phase these out (see Castle 1980).

While the 1974–9 Labour Government sought to reduce the influence of established groups such as the BMA by bringing in groups that were traditionally neglected, particularly trade unions, the Government which replaced them in 1979 was hostile to all such groups – especially the trade unions. The incoming Prime Minister, Margaret Thatcher, was committed to political liberalism and saw the close relationship which ministries had with special interest groups as a threat to the direct relationship with and accountability to citizens. As part of her drive to make government more efficient and more accountable, she launched a cull of government-funded advisory bodies. In health this cull included a network of advisory bodies which had been set up in 1948 to provide advice to the Minister and Ministry on health issues. The Central Health Services Committee, which articulated a range of interests, was abolished, together with four specialist groups, though committees representing doctors and nurses/midwives were retained.

Box 4.4   Reorganising the delivery of health care:
Working for Patients (Department of Health 1989,
see Lawson 1993)

Historical context   During the 1987 general election, the NHS had
been an issue that enabled the Labour Party to make some, but
not sufficient, inroads into the Conservative lead in the opinion
polls. After the election, the Prime Minister appointed a radical
Conservative (John Moores) as Secretary of State to reform the
NHS. However, during the autumn of 1987 there was continued
critical media coverage of the NHS 'funding crisis'.

Process   When interviewed for a BBC TV *Panorama* programme
in January 1988, Thatcher announced a review of the NHS. This
review was 'in-house', including ministers and advisers such as Sir
Roy Griffiths (see Box 2.4). The Prime Minister was committed to
moving from a 'politicised' health service collectively funded from
general taxation to an independent NHS funded through insurance contributions. Griffiths drew attention to the risk that such
a shift could transfer costs to industry, as well as the way it would
enhance trade unions' bargaining power over fringe benefits such
as health insurance.

Outcome   The Review adopted the ideas of an American economist, Alain Enthoven, with funding from general taxation being
allocated through a managed market in which purchasers could
'buy' services from different providers. In January 1989 the
Secretary of State, Kenneth Clarke, published the White Paper
Working for Patients and the enabling legislation was quickly
passed (National Health Service and Community Care Act 1990).
During this period the profession was reduced to the status of an
outsider group and was forced to attack the Government publicly
in the 1992 general election campaign, signalling the loss of its
privileged insider status.

Despite retaining some professional advisory groups, the
Conservative health ministers did not routinely consult the medical
profession over major issues. This arm's-length relationship was
evident in the major reform of health care initiated in 1989. As we
note in box 4.4, for the first time since the 1940s the profession had
no in-put into the planning of major health policy.

In the 1970s and 1980s the role and influence of the medical profession over policy making was progressively reduced. In the late 1970s the profession had to compete with the influence of the trade unions in the Labour Government, while in the 1980s the Conservative Government treated the profession as a specialist interest group that, if necessary, could be consulted and placated but not co-opted into the policy process.

The 1990s and 2000s: from government to governance

Following the Thatcherite assault on the public sector in the 1980s, there were significant changes in the management and nature of the public sector and policy making including:

- *A shift from government to governance* As we noted in chapter 3, the policy and financial crises of the late 1970s precipitated attempts at increasing the efficiency and effectiveness of public services by introducing private-sector managerial techniques and moving to a more entrepreneurial approach to government activities. These were designed to 'promote *competition* between service providers. They *empower* citizens by pushing control out of bureaucracy, into the community. They measure the performance of their agencies, focusing not on inputs but on *outcomes*. They are driven by their goals – their *missions* . . . They redefine their clients as *customers* and offer them choices' (Osborne and Gaebler 1992: 19–20 cited in Rhodes 1997: 49). Such developments changed the nature of government from a central controlling authority to an enabling one – relying not only on a range of public and private bodies but also on citizens for the achievement of its aims and objectives. Thus governance involves a broadening of participation; a shift from control to partnership and a duty for citizens to participate responsibly (see Rhodes 1997: 46–60 for a discussion of the different uses of governance).
- *The development of hyper-innovation and the replacement of the club culture* Moran (2003) noted that the policy crisis of the 1970s was accompanied by an institutional crisis. This undermined the traditional club culture with its emphasis on informal relations within an elite core of decision makers and the self-regulation of institutions such as the medical profession. The change involved a shift from 'informality, reliance on tacit knowledge acquired by insiders by virtue of their insider status, autonomy from public scrutiny and accountability . . . [to] standardization and formality

. . . the provision of systematic information accessible both to insiders and outsiders . . . reporting mechanisms that offer the chance of public control . . . shifts to formality and hierarchy in organization, the expansion of audit into ambitious systems of surveillance' (Moran 2003: 7). This new system involved the continual search for modernisation, i.e. more innovative ways of delivering services. It also represented a major challenge to elites such as the medical profession for whom the move to stand- ardisation and the shift to more formal explicit regulation (which we discuss below) 'threatens their independence from popular control' (Moran 2003: 8).

These changes had a major impact on health policy formation, increasing the importance of health policy and the NHS as the site of new developments in the public sector:

• *Key role of the Department of Health* In the 1990s John Major as Prime Minister reversed Margaret Thatcher's attempt to restrain health expenditure and the Labour government which succeeded him agreed to increase health expenditure to match the OECD average. As we noted in chapter 3, Derek Wanless (2002) esti- mated health expenditure in the UK would rise from £68 billion in 2002/3 to between £154 and £184 billion in 2022/3. The impor- tance of health is not just reflected in its budget but also in its lead role in policy making.
• *Health policy as a leading area of innovation* Many of the key approaches to new forms of governance and regulation have been tested out in the NHS through its modernisation agenda. In 1997 the White Paper *The New NHS: Modern, Dependable* introduced a raft of innovations including clinical governance. This was a new system of regulation in which clinical practice was subject to formal, external regulation. As we noted in chapter 2, in this system, encoded knowledge in the form of guidelines was to replace the use of tacit knowledge as the basis of both policy and clinical decision making. Moreover the performance of clinicians and organisa- tions was subject to inspection, audit and public reporting (see especially chapters in Pickering and Thompson 2003, Alaszewski 2003 and Flynn 2002). In addition, the Department of Health was at the forefront of developing partnerships with the private sector, such as Private Finance Initiatives, to build new hospitals, and has developed a range of policies which provide patients with informa- tion on, and choice between, alternative facilities.

In the 1990s and 2000s, there was a major shift in policy making. Central policy makers instigated a programme of reform that enhanced their ability to control and regulate. The audit culture, evident in reforms such as clinical governance, was designed to increase public trust, knowledge and involvement in the provision of health care (Brown 2008a).

Supplementing expert knowledge with lay consultation

Alongside the development of evidence-based decision making has been an increased emphasis on engaging individuals and groups outside established policy communities through consultation. This commitment to consultation means that the public and patients should be engaged and involved in all processes involved in health from the creation of new knowledge, through the making of policy to the delivery of health and social care. For example, the Research for Patient Benefit Programme funded by the Department of Health specifies that all the research it funds should have patient and public involvement: 'Through Patient and Public Involvement (PPI), people are active partners in the research process by, for example, advising on a research project, assisting in the design of a project, or in carrying out the research, rather than being the subjects of research' (National Institute for Health Research n.d.).

This commitment to consultation underpins the Department's policy making and there is a programme of consultation whose purpose was defined in the following way: 'Consultations are an opportunity for stakeholders and the wider public to contribute to Department of Health policies' (Department of Health 2007).

In the run-up to the 2001 election, ministers decided to issue a major statement on the development of the NHS in the form of an *NHS Plan* (Department of Health 2000a). As preparation for this they engaged in a large-scale consultation that took the form of a listening exercise. The Plan listed the top ten features the public wanted to see, and the first two were fairly expected – more staff and shorter waiting lists – but the third was more surprising: those involved in the consultation wanted the Government to bring back matrons, senior nurses with overall responsibility for nursing and cleaning in traditional hospitals, and we discuss the Secretary of State's response in box 4.5.

In April 2011 the Government decided to initiate another major consultation exercise around plans to reform the NHS, making General Practitioners responsible for most of the local funding of

---

Box 4.5   Alan Milburn and the Modern Matron

Historical context   In the late 1990s Alan Milburn wanted to engage the public in the modernisation of the NHS. In the run-up to the 2001 general election he initiated a large-scale public consultation that fed into *The NHS Plan* (Department of Health 2000a).

Process   Large-scale public consultation using all available technology such as the web, and focus groups of recent users of the NHS, run by the Office of Public Management, who also consulted organisations representing patients.

Participants   152,000 members of the public wrote in, and the other forms of consultation developed a substantial body of information about different interest groups and their concerns.

Policy outcomes   The public response was summarised into 'ten top things that the public want'. These mainly concerned having high-quality accessible services, but the third aspect appeared to challenge the reform agenda and was to bring back a post that predates the NHS – the hospital matron. The plan resolved the tension by creating an oxymoron, the 'Modern Matron' who would have the 'authority to get basics right on the ward' and, in particular, to ensure 'clean wards' (Department of Health 2000a: 12).

---

services. In announcing a two-month pause in the legislative process, the Government promised to 'to "listen and engage" with those with concerns about the NHS reforms' (National Health Executive 2011). However, both the timing and the form of the pause and the associated consultation exercise indicate that this was more about political expediency than about engaging the public in policy making. The consultation was taking place late in the political process, indeed as the legislation that was to give substance to the proposed reforms was being considered by Parliament. The consultation resolved political tensions in the Coalition Government and also enabled it to delay decisions on the reforms until after crucial local elections and the referendum of electoral reform in May 2011. There appeared to be no clear structure to the consultation. A consultation in 2010 on the Department's health business plan and its proposal to change the ways in which the Department assessed the performance of the

NHS included a template for responses, with key questions such as: 'Impact Indicators: In bringing together the high level outcomes from the three separate frameworks, have we ended up with a coherent set of indicators that gives a helpful overview of our performance?' (Department of Health 2010e). The National Health Executive statement announcing the pause and inviting comments on the 2011 reforms included only a very general invitation to comment: 'Tell us what you think at opinion@nationalhealthexecutive.com' (National Health Executive 2011).

Comment

As you will have noted from reading chapters 2, 3 and 4 there have been two separate strands in the development of health policy in Britain. Issues relating to the funding and delivery of health care are highly complex and therefore require systems which can access and utilise sophisticated knowledge. At the same time, the delivery of health care has implications and impacts at one time or another on all the citizens in the United Kingdom, and therefore their active involvement in health policy making has become important. If the knowledge and perceptions of experts and non-experts were similar, then these two aspects of policy making could be complementary strands. However, as we noted in the preface and will expand on in the next chapter, experts and lay people use knowledge in different ways. Experts build up stores of generalisable knowledge which can be used for a variety of purposes including making policies. Individuals living their everyday lives are more concerned with practical knowledge which they build up through experience and use as a guide for immediate action (Alaszewski and Brown 2007). Thus experts and lay people are likely to have very different ways of framing issues. Such differences cannot be resolved by technical processes such as the collection of more information but have to be resolved by the social and political processes which we will consider in more depth in the remainder of this book.

KEY POINTS

- A major change in the environment of policy making took place in the 1980s and 1990s. The traditional informal club culture of UK government was replaced by a more formal system emphasising openness and accountability through the provision of quantitative data on performance. Traditional elites such as the medical profession have had to adjust to this changed environment.

- This change reflected the changing status of the Ministry/Department of Health. In the 1940s and 1950s the Ministry was a minor department with a limited budget, little political influence and restricted policy development. By the 2000s the Department was one of the most politically important, with a rapidly expanding budget and a lead role in policy and service innovation.
- In the 1940s the medical profession was co-opted into policy making and, through backstairs networks, played a key role. In the 1970s other challenging and repressed interests were given increasing voice. The medical profession clearly remains an important participant in the policy process but no longer has the dominant veto power of the 1940s and 1950s.
- The Department of Health has broadened participation in health policy making. While the policy core of ministers and their advisers continues to play a key role in policy making, there is a commitment to broadening participation through consulting individuals and groups outside the traditional health policy community. Such consultation can be relatively tokenistic, an expediency to deal with a political crisis – for example, the consultation that accompanied the two-month pause in the legislation to implement the 2011 NHS reforms. However, it can be more serious and systematic as in the listening exercise which preceded *The NHS Plan* in 2000.

5

The pressure of events: disasters, inquiries and the dynamics of blame

AIMS

To consider the impact of events such as disasters on health policy making, and the ways in which such events restrict the scope for rational policy making.

OBJECTIVES

- To examine the ways in which disasters disrupt the rational approach to policy making in which decisions based upon evidence gained from past events are designed to manage the future
- To examine the ways in which disasters disrupt the predictable relationship between past, present and future – undermining policy makers' control of events and replacing risk with uncertainty
- To consider the ways in which disasters threaten established order whereby, in attempting to regain control and re-establish trust, policy makers need to invoke external authority in the form of independent inquiries
- To analyse the role of inquiries as emotional catharsis and in finding out what happened and allocating blame
- To examine how and why disasters and related inquiries have become central to policy making in health.

In chapters 1 to 4 we examined why rationality was important in policy making and how core policy makers such as ministers and their advisers strived to achieve rational policy making by accessing appropriate knowledge and expertise and consulting over policy.

These core policy makers aim to control and improve the future by using knowledge gained from the scientific study of past events. Such rationality needs time and resources, but when things go wrong and disasters happen there is pressure for immediate action, and in this chapter we consider the impact of this pressure on policy making.

5.1 The increasing importance of disasters in modern societies

Disasters are not a new phenomenon. Premodern states had to cope with natural disasters such as harvest failure and epidemic disease. An epidemic of bubonic plague (Black Death) killed approximately a third of the European population between 1348 and 1350. These states also had to deal with man-made disasters such as military defeats or revolts by elites or peasants. They struggled to restore traditional order using contemporary knowledge – especially religious knowledge – to understand and respond to these events.

As governments developed their modern forms and rationales, they continued to be affected by traditional disasters, as well as new ones linked to failures in emerging welfare services. Scandals in late eighteenth and early nineteenth centuries around publicly funded asylums for lunatics, such as Royal Bethlem in London and York Asylum, exposed major shortcomings and stimulated a reform movement. In 1813 Godfrey Higgins, a magistrate, investigated the York Asylum and uncovered mistreatment and financial irregularities. Unable to get action to remedy the problems, he informed the press, but to prevent a full investigation the staff burnt down part of the building, killing four patients and destroying incriminating records. This stimulated a Parliamentary inquiry into conditions in asylums (Jones 1972: 64–73). Similarly, a number of the workhouses established by the 1834 Poor Law Amendment Act (see chapter 1 and box 1.4) were exposed as having inhumane conditions in which paupers suffered physical and sexual abuse and starvation (Rees 2001: 61–2).

In the twentieth century, disasters have become increasingly important for a number of reasons (see Alaszewski and Burgess 2007).

- *The increasing incidence of man-made disasters* Perrow has argued that modern societies are based on high-risk systems – with tightly coupled ones (possessing little room for error) making accidents inevitable, even normal (Perrow 1999: 4). The development of technologies such as nuclear power, nuclear weapons and genetic engineering has created new potential for catastrophic disasters to affect vast swathes of people and future generations (1999: 307). Given the increasing importance of technology in health care, normal accidents are also apparent in this domain. At the Kent and Canterbury Hospital, 90,000 cervical screening slides were re-examined after evidence emerged that screeners had missed hundreds of cancers. The mistakes resulted in 'avoidable deaths' of at least eight women, thirty women undergoing avoidable hysterectomies, financial compensation for at least three women, and an apology from the Trust's chief executive. However, an external review by the Royal College of Pathologists found that errors were within the expected range and 'acceptable mistakes' affected 1.6 per cent of cases (*BBC News* 1999).

- *Lack of public confidence and trust in government* As we noted in chapter 1, governments in modern democracies claim that they act in the interest of all citizens and that their policies are designed to enhance welfare and protect wellbeing for all citizens. Health and welfare systems seek the confidence and trust of the public and patients – in the case of the NHS through ensuring it is a 'high trust' organisation (Department of Health 2000b: 56 – we return to the issue of trust in chapter 7). Disasters such as deaths from hospital-acquired infections highlight the ways in which health care can harm rather than protect citizens. For example, between 2004 and 2006, an outbreak of *Clostridium difficile* (*C. diff*) in NHS hospitals in West Kent infected at least 1,176 patients and contributed to 345 deaths (Carvel 2007). The media coverage of the incident was highly critical and included headlines such as 'Cover-ups, lies and the cynical conspiracy that let a superbug claim 90 lives' (Clarke 2007). Such coverage of failures can undermine public trust in the government. In the case of BSE (mad cow disease) in the 1990s, the government sought to reassure the public that it was safe to eat British beef. The public was initially willing to accept such reassurances but attitudes changed after the Secretary of State for Health announced evidence that some individuals had acquired a neurological degenerative disease (vCJD) through eating infected beef, and the effects of this are discussed in box 5.1.
- *The need to allocate blame for the failure to identify and prevent risk* As Douglas (1990) has argued, the concept of risk is increasingly used in the same way as sin is in religious societies – to identify

---

Box 5.1   The BSE disaster (Reilly 1999: 128–45)

Context   In 1984, cattle in England were infected by a new disease identified in 1986 by the Ministry of Agriculture, Fisheries and Food (MAFF) as Bovine Spongiform Encephalopathy (BSE) – referred to in the popular press as 'mad cow disease'. There was a possibility that in the 1980s infected beef had entered the human food chain. Throughout the decade, there was a tension amongst policy makers between those concerned with farming and the production of cheap food, especially MAFF, and those concerned with public health and the safety of food, especially the Department of Health and Social Security.

Representing British beef as safe   Mainstream media coverage of BSE started in 1987 with the headline in the *Sunday Telegraph*: 'Incurable disease wiping out our dairy cows' (25 October 1987). Policy makers associated with food production initially took the lead in providing advice and guidance for the media. Scientific advisers took the view that there was no evidence that BSE could affect humans. Key policy makers emphasised that eating beef was safe. For example, in January 1990, the Government's Chief Vet stated in an interview, published in *The Times*, that human infection was a remote possibility. Subsequently, the Chief Medical Officer stated that 'There is no risk associated with eating British beef [and] it's safe to eat'. To reinforce the message, MAFF staged an event in which the press were able to photograph the Minister, John Gummer, eating a beef-burger and appearing to feed one to his four-year-old daughter. The initial media coverage peaked in 1990, and was strongly influenced by the 'beef is safe' representation.

Collapse of the strategy   There were counterclaims by microbiologists Helen Grant and Richard Lacey, but officials represented these critics as mavericks. In March 1996 new scientific evidence forced the Secretary of State for Health, Stephen Dorrell, to announce in Parliament deaths from a new variant of Creutzfeld-Jakob Disease (vCJD), a degenerative disease affecting the human brain and central nervous system, and that this disease was probably caused by eating beef infected with BSE. Dorrell subsequently expressed regret that prior to the statement he had reassured the public that there was 'no conceivable risk' (*BBC News* 2000). The ministerial announcement was greeted with shock by the media, which now emphasised the dangers associated with eating beef and the horror of vCJD.

Audience response to media messages   The Glasgow Media Group monitored public response to BSE in the 1990s. The Group found that mass media were the main source of information. Initially BSE was predominantly viewed as a media scare, another food panic. While participants did not fully trust the Government, they were willing to accept its message about the safety of beef. Following the ministerial announcement, however, attitudes changed dramatically. A sense of shock and uncertainty resulted in a 're-evaluation both of the media as source of critical information and of politicians/government officials as reliable providers of health messages' (Reilly 1999: 137).

(moral) failing and to allocate blame in the context of disasters. This underpins the development of a 'blame culture', in which all harmful events are seen as a product of human agency and every misfortune is someone's fault: 'under the banner of risk reduction, a new blaming system has replaced the former' system based on religion and sin (Douglas 1992: 16). If the media succeed in identifying the 'guilty' party then a disaster becomes a scandal and there is pressure for the guilty to be punished. In the case of the *C. difficile* outbreak mentioned above, the chief executive of the NHS Trust was blamed for 'a conspiracy of secrecy, went on to bare-faced lies and ended with an almighty cover-up of the true extent of the crisis' (Clarke 2007). She was forced to resign, and the Secretary of State, Alan Johnson, blocked her agreed resignation settlement of £400,000.

Disasters threaten the established order and ontological security which can be defined as the collective confidence in the essential stability and predictability of everyday life (Giddens 1990: 92). Threats to this security require some sort of collective response. While the level of harm is clearly important in defining an event as a disaster, other factors are involved – especially the perceived horror and sense of threat stimulated by the event. Given the collective nature of the threat, disasters involve some mechanism which converts private misfortune into public disaster, usually media coverage (see chapter 9).

In private misfortunes, the harm and loss is experienced by those immediately involved. In disasters, the consequences are not restricted to those immediately involved, but through wider coverage spread beyond and imply a broader threat to those not directly concerned. There is a shift in perception which is often described as a 'shock' and such disastrous events are often described as shocking. Underpinning this shock is a shift from seeing the future as essentially predictable and manageable – for example in terms of risk that can be used to define the probability of different outcomes – to viewing the future as uncertain and therefore unmanageable, as the past is no longer seen as a reliable guide to the future (Alaszewski and Coxon 2008). For example the Editor of the *BMJ*, when commenting on the consequences of the events that led to the appointment of the Bristol Royal Infirmary Inquiry, entitled his editorial 'All changed, changed utterly' (Smith 1998).

Such disasters reduce the scope for rational policy making by:

- *Focusing attention on particular unique circumstances and individuals* Rational policy is concerned with creating improvements for the whole population, or general categories of individuals such as young people who misuse drugs, rather than the special and atypical situation of specific victims of a disaster.
- *Concentrating on the present or immediate past* Rational policy deals with imagined situations; it attempts to predict and improve the future. Responding to disasters involves understanding and dealing with real events that have already happened.
- *Creating pressure for immediate action* Rational policy requires time for the collection and interpretation of relevant evidence. Once a disaster is identified, then key decision makers need to be seen to act, immediately taking personal responsibility and leadership, bypassing the normal bureaucratic system. They are also expected to show personal concern, for example by visiting the scene and sympathising with the victims and their suffering. For example, in June 2010, the Prime Minister (David Cameron) and Home Secretary (Theresa May) visited Cumbria two days after the 'horrific events' in which a local man randomly shot and killed people. The Prime Minister stated that 'I wanted to come here to show [that] the Government wanted to listen, wanted to show how much it cares about what happened here' (Number 10 2010).
- *Compelling decision makers to act in the media spotlight in an emotionally charged situation* Rational policy requires both time and space within which decision makers can make objective judgements and the best decisions. Disasters create a 'media frenzy' (see chapter 9) in which the mass media highlight the suffering of the victims and seek to allocate blame for this suffering. This denies policy makers both the time and space they want, due to pressure to make decisions as they want to show they are taking quick action.

- *Undermining the public acceptability of policies* Disasters indicate the failure of existing policies and the knowledge and expertise on which these policies are based. As Perrow (1999) noted in his analysis of the Three Mile Island disaster in the USA, the policy of building such nuclear power stations was based on expert risk analyses that a failure was a very unlikely and rare event that would only occur once every 300 years. The disaster indicated to the public that such failures were possible and that, since experts predicted that they would almost never happen, experts were fallible.

Policy makers can respond to disasters by trying to adapt quickly and develop policies, and in chapter 9 we discuss the case of the 1991 Dangerous Dogs Act. However, one well-established way of defusing the situation is to appoint an inquiry, buying time but at the same time showing that policy makers care and are taking the situation seriously.

5.2 Responding to disaster: the impact of inquiries on policy

Admission of failure

Though inquiries are not limited to disasters, the appointment of an independent inquiry indicates serious failure and that the normal policy-making process cannot deal with the situation. Since disasters tend to undermine confidence in the government: 'The main outcome [of an independent investigation] must be to increase public confidence' (National Health Service London 2010a: 18). One way of doing this is to exploit the authority, expertise and trustworthiness of independent experts, especially judges: 'the deployment by politicians of the judges' status and credibility to defuse matters which those politicians feel they can neither safely ignore nor tackle by normal political and parliamentary methods' (Drewry 1996: 369). But this means that such inquiries are intrinsically difficult to control and their outcomes unpredictable.

Ministers try to control the findings of inquiries through selecting their chairs and members and specifying their terms of reference. However, given the status and autonomy of inquiry committees since the late 1960s, they have tended to overstep their terms of reference. This development can be seen in box 5.2 which shows the shift from a deferential and protective approach to investigation to a more critical one in two inquiries investigating allegations at the end of the 1960s. The Regional Inquiries into allegations of abuse of elderly

Box 5.2   The shift to more critical inquiries in the late
           1960s

Historical context   In the 1960s there was substantial investment
in hospital building, mostly new acute hospitals but also some
hospitals for long-stay patients who were elderly, learning disabled
or mentally ill. There was a growing criticism of long-stay hospitals (see Jones and Fowles 1984). In November 1965, *The Times*
published a letter by Barbara Robb and her colleagues alleging
maltreatment of older patients in mental hospitals, noting a lack
of response by the Ministry of Health to such allegations, and
inviting those who had encountered malpractice to contact them.
In 1967 Barbara Robb, acting on behalf of AEGIS (Aid for the
Elderly in Government Institutions), published *Sans Everything*
(Robb 1967) – claiming to provide evidence of massive corrup-
tion and cruelty in NHS hospitals. In August 1967 the *News of the
World* published a statement by a nursing assistant (named XY)
at Ely Hospital, Cardiff, alleging that some staff were sadistic,
patients were beaten regularly, and that the senior managers and
doctors did not care.

The Inquiries   The Minister of Health, Kenneth Robinson,
decided, in view of public concern, to appoint Inquiries. In the
case of the Robb allegation, the Regional Hospital Boards undertook the inquiries. The investigation into the allegations at Ely
Hospital was undertaken by an independent inquiry team chaired
by Geoffrey Howe, then a barrister. Its terms of reference were
specifically limited to the allegations published in the *News of the
World* and the 'situation in the wards in the hospital at the current
time' (National Health Service 1969: 1–2). The Inquiry had no
power to summon witnesses and a request by the Inquiry team to
have a solicitor to help them to organise and process evidence was
refused.

Outcome   The Regional Inquiries into Robb's allegations refuted
her claims including those made in 'the Diary of a Nobody' which
was part of *Sans Everything*. They concluded that her book was a
'serious distortion of the facts' (National Health Service 1968: 27).
The Inquiries did not recommend any major changes in policy,
and in his response to their report the Minister indicated that he
felt Robb's publication was an abuse of free speech (Martin with

Evans 1984: 5). In contrast, the Ely Inquiry concluded that 'the situation at Ely has proved to be sufficiently disturbing to make XY's concerns well justified. It is a matter of speculation how long the situation would have persisted had it not been for XY's communication to the *News of the World*.' The Inquiry exceeded its terms of reference, criticising not only the hospital and its wards but also the lack of leadership provided by those NHS bodies responsible for funding and supervising the hospital: 'we have concluded that there is a clear need, within the present structure of the health service, for some system of inspection of a hospital like Ely, which will ensure that those responsible for its management are made aware of what needs to be done to bring it up to the standard which the Minister aims to achieve' (National Health Service 1969: 115–17).

patients dismissed the allegations as ill founded (National Health Service 1968), while the Inquiry into allegations of abuses at Ely Hospital in Cardiff not only found the allegations proven but went on to criticise the NHS management and, by implication, central government (National Health Service 1969).

Finding the truth: the rationality of hindsight

Inquiries are appointed to find out what happened and how it can be prevented from happening again. Lord Salmon, in the Royal Commission on Tribunals of Inquiry, stated their role was 'to take and direct all necessary searching investigations and to produce the witnesses in order to arrive at the truth' (Her Majesty's Government 1966: para 28). The independent investigation into the treatment of BM, a substance-misusing mentally ill person who on 15 September 2006 stabbed Tom-Louis Easton to death, described the purpose of the Inquiry in the following way:

> The purpose of an Independent Investigation is to thoroughly review the care and treatment received by the patient in order to establish the lessons to be learnt, to minimise the possibility of a reoccurrence of similar events, and to make recommendations for the delivery of Health Services in the future, incorporating what can be learnt from a robust analysis of the individual case. (National Health Service London 2010b: 6)

Inquiries try to establish the facts. In cases such as Ely where the evidence about harm is disputed, the first step is to examine allegations of harm to see whether they are substantiated (see NHS 1969: 8–56). Similarly, the Inquiry into the management of the care of children receiving complex cardiac surgical services at the Bristol Royal Infirmary between 1984 and 1995 (Bristol Royal Infirmary Inquiry 2001) commissioned an expert review of mortality in the service. This review focused on the period 1991–5, for which there was comparable national data, and concluded that during this period (allowing for variations in case mix) there were 30 to 35 more deaths than there should have been at Bristol Royal Infirmary (Spiegelhalter et al. 2000: 3).

The next step is to identify the causes of the harm. Where there is a major focal event, such as a murder, inquiries tend to focus on the preceding events and decisions in order to identify the fatal flaws. The investigation into the treatment of BM first established an overall chronology of the life of BM before developing a time-line of events leading up to the key event: BM's killing of Tom-Louis Easton. The investigation explored the causes of the disaster using a Root Cause Analysis Fishbone (National Health Service London 2010b: 31–81 and 104–19). Similarly, the Inquiry into the killing of Jonathan Zito included 'The Christopher Clunis story' (Ritchie Inquiry 1994: 7–104), reconstructing events, especially those from July 1987 when Clunis first attended a London hospital for treatment for his mental health to December 1992 when he killed Jonathan Zito. The Inquiry concluded that 'the problem was cumulative; it was one failure or missed opportunity on top of another. As a result of these numerous failures and omissions by a number of people and agencies [no effective action was taken to prevent Jonathan Zito's death]' (Ritchie Inquiry 1994: 105).

The role of hindsight is evident in the ways in which the Inquiry identified phenomena whose significance only became evident in the light of future events. Christopher Clunis's early interest in knives became noteworthy in the context of his later delusions and violence (Ritchie Inquiry 1994: 8). From this perspective, various professionals minimised the significance of Clunis's later use of knives and thus 'failed' to recognise it as a warning sign (Ritchie Inquiry 1994: 26).

From analyses of unique sequences of events in highly atypical situations inquiries are invited to generalise about the underlying general causes of harm, and make recommendations for changes in systems and practices designed to prevent a repetition of disasters. Such recommendations often involve the development of more effective systems for identifying and managing risk. The Ritchie Inquiry (1994) singled out the repeated failure of practitioners from a range of services to effectively assess the danger posed by Christopher Clunis. It recommended that mental health patients who had a history of violence should have formal aftercare plans which included 'an assessment . . . as to whether the patient's propensity for violence presents any risk to his own health or safety or to the protection of the public' (Ritchie Inquiry 1994: 111). However, there is also recognition in some reports that the final disaster could not have been predicted or prevented: 'The Independent Investigation Panel consider [sic] that the tragic homicide of Tom-Louis Easton by Mr BM could not have been predicted. The care and treatment of Mr BM could have been better . . . There was no single cause of the homicide other than the fact that Mr BM did have a serious mental illness for which he was being treated' (National Health Service London 2010b: 87). This conclusion did not stop the investigation team making recommendations for service improvements.

It is possible to take an overview of a number of inquiry reports to identify common causes of different disasters. The Department of Health and Social Security (1982) published an overview of child abuse inquiries identifying the systemic failures of health and social care organisations, such as failures to identify warning signs, to communicate and to collaborate. Turner and Pidgeon (1997), undertaking a study of man-made disasters based on a review of eighty-four disaster and accident reports published by the UK government over eleven years (1965–75), similarly identified the ways in which senior managers disregarded warnings and insulated themselves from reality.

However, despite repeated inquiries and syntheses of evidence in areas such as child abuse and homicides by former mental-health patients, there is little evidence of successful prevention. As in other spheres, the highly formalised micro 'risk management of everything' has no clear relationship to improved outcomes (Power 2007). Consequently, new inquiries tend to identify the same failings as previous ones, if sometimes denouncing them in ever more strident terms.

Providing emotional catharsis

Contemporary forensic inquiries also have a cathartic function. They can be used for 'pacifying communal feelings' (Blom-Cooper 1996: 59), as in the case of the Aberfan disaster when, in 1966, a coal tip slid onto a village killing 144 people, 116 of them children (Aberfan n.d.).

The inquiry can serve a cathartic function by providing survivors and victims' families with a forum for their grief and an opportunity to listen to witnesses. Recent inquiries have been concerned to listen to victims and to give them a voice. The Inquiry into the retention of organs and tissue at Alder Hey Hospital in Liverpool invited all parents involved to complete a questionnaire that encouraged them 'to say in their own words how they felt about the death of their child'. Forty-three representative parents were invited to give oral evidence. All parents were offered counselling if and when they felt they needed it (House of Commons 2001: 9). The Inquiry into paediatric surgery at Bristol Royal Infirmary accepted that an important part of its function was to enable those parents whose children had been harmed to develop an understanding of what happened: 'A Public Inquiry cannot turn back the clock. It can . . . offer an opportunity for those touched by events, in our case Bristol, to be heard and listen to others. Through this process can come understanding' (Bristol Royal Infirmary Inquiry 2001: Foreword).

In modern psychological jargon, inquiries can provide *closure* for those affected by the disaster. Thus the investigation into the treatment of Mr BM expressed the hope 'that this Report will help to address any issues that have remained unresolved to-date' (National Health Service London 2010b: 5). The report contained condolences to the family of Tom-Louis Easton and a tribute to him from his family and friends.

One way in which those affected by the disaster can achieve closure is if the inquiry allocates blame and the guilty parties are named, shamed and punished.

Allocating blame

Generally speaking, inquiries claim that they are focusing on system failures so that the systems can be improved to prevent reoccurrence. They typically state that their role is not to allocate blame. The Ashworth Inquiry stated that: 'A public inquiry which is inquisitorial is aimed primarily at establishing the truth rather than proving guilt or innocence' (National Health Service 1999: para. 1.4.2). Similarly the Inquiry into the killing of Jonathan Zito by Christopher Clunis stated that: 'We do not single out just one person, service or agency for particular blame' (Ritchie Inquiry 1994: 105). Despite these disclaimers, inquiries do allocate blame. The Inquiry into Zito's death scrutinised and judged the actions of those involved in the events leading up to the killing. The Inquiry noted Dr Michael Roth, a Clinical Assistant, felt that Clunis's attempts to stab people did not indicate he was a dangerous person. With the benefit of hindsight, they judged he was wrong: 'We feel that Dr Roth's view was given with the best interests of his patient at heart, but we feel his view was misguided and such a superficial view can ultimately lead to serious danger to the patient or to the public or both' (Ritchie Inquiry 1994: 26).

The Inquiry into paediatric surgery at Bristol Royal Infirmary focused on the systemic failures within the service and the hospital. The Inquiry argued that the staff at the hospital had collectively failed to protect the vulnerable children in their care. It was a story of 'people who cared greatly about human suffering, and were dedicated and well-motivated. Sadly, some lacked insight and their behaviour was flawed. Many failed to communicate with each other, and to work together for the interests of their patients. There was a lack of leadership and of teamwork' (The Bristol Royal Infirmary Inquiry 2001: Synopsis). The Inquiry identified a '"a club culture"; an imbalance of power, with too much control in the hands of a few individuals' (2001: Synopsis).

Having identified the importance of disasters and associated inquiries in policy making, in the final section of this chapter we consider the increasing importance of inquiries in health policy making.

5.3 The increasing importance of disasters and inquiries in health policy making

The absence of disasters in the early years of the NHS (1948–1968)

In the early years of the NHS there were independent inquiries indicating the existence of problems which routine policy making could not deal with. These issues related mainly to relationships with the medical profession, especially over the terms and conditions of doctors' employment (see chapter 1, especially box 1.5) and the overall cost of the NHS (see chapters 1 and 3 for discussions of the Guillebaud Inquiry). Such inquiries generally did not focus on failures in service deliveries or incidents that caused major harm to service users and others. One exception, which we describe in box 5.3, was the Royal Commission on the Law relating to Mental Illness and Mental Deficiency, and even in this case the claimed disaster was more of a catalyst than a prime cause of the Inquiry (Alaszewski 1983: 227–31; Jones 1972: 283–320).

It is possible but unlikely that the absence of disasters and inquiries

Box 5.3 The Royal Commission on the Law relating to Mental Illness and Mental Deficiency (1957)

Context When the NHS was created in 1948, institutions such as former lunatic asylums and mental deficiency colonies were incorporated into the NHS as long-stay hospitals. These institutions continued to work within the framework of Victorian and Edwardian mental health legislation. The people being treated within these hospitals had a special legal status and their treatment and continued confinement was regulated by the Board of Control which became a Division of the Ministry of Health. The National Council for Civil Liberties (1951) published a pamphlet (*50,000 Outside the Law*) which focused on the ways in which individuals detained in mental deficiency hospitals were deprived of their civil liberties and exploited. Concerns about the treatment of patients with mental illness and mental deficiency were raised by MPs in a critical debate in Parliament in February 1954.

The Government response: the Royal Commission The Ministry of Health recognised that major changes were taking place within the care of people with mental illness and learning disabilities, but that the Ministry did not have the capacity to review current policies and legislation. Given the sensitive nature of the issue, the Minister decided to appoint a high-level expert committee, a Royal Commission. The Royal Commission received a memorandum from the Chairman and the Senior Medical Officer of the Board of Control recommending the abolition of the existing legalistic framework as it was hindering the development of more progressive community-based services. It was suggested that some legal power needed to be retained, for example when people were in the acute phase of mental illness and were a danger to themselves or others and could not judge their own best interest. Yet in general most people with mental illness and mental deficiency should not be subject to legal controls but be treated as voluntary patients. The Commission accepted these proposals and they formed the basis of its recommendations.

Legal reform The 1959 Mental Health Act implemented the recommendations of the Royal Commission. It provided new legal definitions of different types of mental disorder, specifying that 'promiscuity or other immoral conduct' would not of itself

be regarded as a mental disorder. It specified the narrow range of
circumstances in which individuals with mental disorder could be
legally compelled to have treatment and enabled most people with
mental disorder to be treated voluntarily. It incorporated services
within the mainstream, replacing the 'watchdog' functions of the
Board of Control with Mental Health Review Tribunals.

in the early phase of the NHS indicates that medical and other practitioners did not make mistakes which resulted in preventable harm
and death. It is more likely that a number of factors contributed to
the suppression of evidence of such errors, with preventable injury
and deaths remaining private misfortunes rather becoming public
disasters. The contributing factors included:

- *Institutional protection of medical practitioners and the NHS* In the
  early phase of the NHS, the courts were reluctant to challenge
  medical decisions and the standards which doctors set for their
  own practice (Price 2010). In the case of *Bolam v. Friern Hospital
  Management Committee* (Queens Bench Division 1957), the judge
  established the principle that if a doctor reached the standard of a
  responsible body of medical opinion, he was not negligent, even if
  as a consequence of his action his patient suffered serious harm.
  Collectively the NHS was also protected by Crown immunity.
  Thus inspectorates could advise the NHS on standards, such as
  health and safety, but could not take legal action to enforce standards (Barker and Storey 1992).
- *Health as a political and policy backwater* As we noted in chapters
  1 and 2, following the creation of the NHS in 1948 health policy
  was primarily a matter of low, routine politics, i.e. administering
  health and related services. The Ministry of Health was a civil
  service backwater and the Minister was not necessarily in the
  cabinet. Only in exceptional circumstances – mainly relating to
  conflict with the medical profession, the costs of the service or
  major investment – did health become part of high politics, i.e.
  matters affecting or threatening the whole of the government. As
  we showed in chapter 4, more mundane issues such as standards
  of services were treated as technical matters to be dealt with by the
  medical profession and the Ministry.
- *Limited role of the mass media* In the 1950s and 1960s the role of
  investigative journalism was relatively limited. The media were
  relatively deferential and did not seem interested in criticising the

government over health policy (see chapter 9 for a discussion of the media).

- *Public acceptance* The first generation to use the NHS, especially those from more deprived areas, had experience of the deprivations of the 1930s Depression and the Second World War and the difficulties and costs of accessing health care. This generation appears to have been grateful to accept the benefits of the new service and was therefore relatively uncritical. In a study of three generations of women whose husbands were in unskilled or semi-skilled jobs, the older generation (born mostly in the 1930s) 'did not appear to be efficient and demanding users of services' (Blaxter and Paterson 1982: 195), and they were relatively uncritical of doctors, seeing their GP as 'a family friend who is at the same time an expert' (Blaxter and Paterson 1982: 195).

Disaster and inquiries in the mature NHS

Between 1968 and 1998, disasters and inquiries became established parts of policy making in the NHS, especially in services and areas that were marginal to the mainstream, e.g. services for older people, services for people with mental illness and disability, and child protection services. Only very rarely did disasters in other services – such as the contamination of infusion fluids at Plymouth General Hospital (National Health Service 1972a) – merit an inquiry.

We noted above that the Ely Inquiry (1968–9) took a critical and analytical approach, and its Report (National Health Service 1969) had a major impact on policy for people with learning disabilities. It was the precursor to a series of inquiries into long-stay hospitals. Martin with Evans (1984) lists twenty inquiries between 1968 and 1980 dividing them into:

- *The problems of the old order (1968–1974) Farleigh Hospital* for men with severe learning disabilities over sixteen; allegations of serious violence (National Health Service 1971) *Whittingham Hospital*, a large mental hospital catering mainly for long-stay patients; allegations of ill-treatment, violence, victimisation, maladministration and financial irregularities (National Health Service 1972b)
- *The problems of a changing system (1975–1979) Warlingham Park Hospital*, a mental illness hospital of good reputation; investigation into high number of in- and out-patient suicides during 1974 and 1975 (Croydon Area Health Authority 1976) *Normansfield Hospital*, a learning disability hospital in which the Consultant

had developed an excessively 'safety first' attitude because of his reading of other inquiry reports and his concern about being held responsible for any untoward incident. This provoked a strike in the hospital during which 200 patients with learning disabilities were exposed to serious danger (National Health Service 1978)

- *Unfinished business (1980 onwards) Rampton Hospital*, a special hospital; allegations of large-scale brutality to patients and refusal of staff to adopt new practices (Department of Health and Social Security 1980). The challenges of reforming Rampton are outlined in box 5.4.

Political and social changes underlie the increasing recognition of disasters in long-stay hospitals and the use of inquiries to analyse their causes and recommend changes. The processes that prevented private misfortunes from becoming public disasters were increasingly undermined:

- *Questioning of the institutional protection of medical practitioners and the NHS* In the 1970s and 1980s the courts started challenging medical decisions. For example, in the case of *Whitehouse v. Jordan and another* the trial judge found that Jordan, an obstetrician, had been negligent in the way he conducted delivery by forceps, causing severe brain damage to Stuart Whitehouse, the baby, and awarded £100,000 damages. In this case the Appeal Court over-turned the decision. However, Lord Denning in his judgement clearly expressed anxiety about increasing litigation. He noted that Stuart's parents had tried to turn their private misfortune into a public disaster by campaigning for an inquiry and he warned: 'Take heed of what has happened in the United States. "Medical malpractice" cases there are very worrying, especially as they are tried by juries who have sympathy for the patient and none for the doctor' (Court of Appeal, Civil Division 1980: 10). Despite Lord Denning's warnings, increased public funding, plus the growth of law firms specialising in negligence, meant that the UK was moving in the same direction as the USA. In the 1980s the institutional protection of the NHS was also reduced.
- *Health policy moves into the mainstream* The era of hospital disasters and inquiries started at the same time as Richard Crossman was appointed as Secretary of State for Health and Social Services. This major cabinet-level post indicated that health policy had become a key part of government policy. Crossman and his successors were keen to make a mark and used inquiry reports to initiate

Box 5.4   The Rampton Hospital Inquiry: an iconic hospital scandal (Department of Health and Social Security 1980, and Martin with Evans 1984: 51–7)

Historical context   Special hospitals had a distinctive position and role in the NHS. They provided treatment and special security for patients who were dangerous, were violent or had criminal propensities, and were directly managed by the Department of Health and Social Security. They were in some senses 'flagships' of the traditional institutional system, taking the most challenging patients from other hospitals and providing a highly secure and controlled environment. Given their secrecy, isolation, specialist role and strong culture they were resistant to change and reform. Rampton was a special hospital devoted mainly to the treatment of patients with learning disabilities. In the early 1970s the Hospital Advisory Service and a Department of Health and Social Security-commissioned consultant had undertaken internal reviews and indicated the need for modernisation. In May 1979, Yorkshire Television broadcast 'The secret hospital', alleging 801 cases of brutal treatment of patients by over 100 nurses.

The Government response   The Secretary of State responded to the allegations by referring all cases of alleged abuse to the Director of Public Prosecutions and setting up a Review Team led by a retired local government manager, Sir John Boyton. The Team identified a highly isolated institution which lacked leadership, both from the Department of Health and Social Security and locally from the medical staff and managers. Nurses used their membership of the Prison Officers Association to resist modernisation and change, especially any reform of their 14-hour working day. The reluctance of other hospitals to accept Rampton patients meant that there was a backlog of discharges, contributing to overcrowding.

Reform of the special hospitals   The Review Team initiated a process that resulted in substantial change in the special hospitals. While nurses at Rampton continued to resist change, the Department of Health and Social Security appointed a medical director and a Review Board to initiate and manage modernisation. Over time special hospitals were absorbed into the NHS mainstream, e.g. in 1989 the Department of Health created the Special

Hospitals Authority that distanced it from their day-to-day management, and in 1996 their management was transferred to local
NHS Trusts. The development of regional medium secure units
created a link between the modernised high secure services and
the low secure community-based services (see Nottinghamshire
Healthcare NHS n.d.).

change. For example, in his diaries, Crossman (1977) described
how his civil servants advised him to minimise the impact of the
Ely Hospital Report by only publishing the concluding chapter.Yet
he disregarded their advice, seeing the Report as an opportunity
to initiate change – creating a hospital inspectorate to act as his
'eyes and ears' and establishing a working party to review policy
for people with learning disabilities.

* *Increasing investigative role of the mass media* Martin with Evans
(1984) identified the key role of the print and television media in
identifying disasters. He noted that the professional media provided a forum for staff, who were often the first people to identify
problems and publicise them, i.e. whistle-blowers. Newspapers
and television then played a key role in converting local incidents
into national scandals (as in the case of nurse XY at Ely Hospital,
discussed in box 5.2). Television documentaries also had a major
impact, as in the case of Yorkshire Television's exposé of Rampton
Hospital, 'The secret hospital'.

* *More critical and active public* The second generation to use
the NHS were born in the late 1940s and 1950s, the so-called
'Baby Boom' generation. They grew up during a period of relative prosperity, with the full benefits of the welfare state. This
generation appears to have very much higher expectations of
the NHS. Blaxter noted that the response of the Baby Boomers
to services were more varied than those of their mothers. Some
Baby Boomers adopted the relatively uncritical attitude of their
mothers but still expected responsive services, but most adopted
a more active consumerist approach (Blaxter and Paterson
1982: 195). This more critical approach to public services was
reflected at collective as well as individual levels. In the 1960s and
1970s there was a growth in the number and activity of groups
representing the users of public services, as we will discuss in
chapter 6.

Disasters in core areas and the routinisation of inquiries
(1988–present)

Since 1988 the scope of inquiries has broadened beyond the marginal, problem areas of health and social care to core services.

- *Further inquiries in problem services* Most long-stay hospitals have shut, although inquiries continued in those that survived. Sir Louis Blom Cooper conducted an inquiry into Ashworth special hospital following a television documentary claiming staff had beaten a patient to death. His report identified a brutal, dehumanising regime (National Health Service 1992).
  As services shifted to the community, so did disasters such as the killing of Jonathan Zito by Christopher Clunis, and related inquiries (Ritchie Inquiry 1994). Disasters and inquiries also continued in the child protection services. Most of these related to failures of services to protect children, e.g. Victoria Climbié (Laming 2003). There were also inquiries into new aspects of child protection, cases in which social workers and others appeared to be excessively cautious and removed children from their parents when the evidence of harm was contested, as we show in box 9.5 that discusses the Cleveland and Orkney Inquiries.
- *Inquiries within mainstream services such as general hospitals and general practice* These have tended to focus on the harmful practices and behaviours of specific practitioners and the system failures which meant their harmful activities were not identified at an early stage. There were inquiries into Beverley Allitt, a nurse who deliberately injured and killed children at Grantham and Kesteven General Hospital (Clothier Inquiry 1994), and Harold Shipman, a general practitioner who was convicted of killing 15 of his elderly patients but probably killed at least 260 (Shipman Inquiry 2002: para 14.2).
- *Inquiries and disasters in teaching hospitals* These hospitals are meant to be centres of excellence, train future doctors in best practice and set the highest standards for other services. Box 5.5 describes two major interrelated disasters and inquiries which occurred at Bristol Royal Infirmary and Alder Hey Children's Hospital in Liverpool.
- *Public health: protecting and reassuring the public* After 1974, health policy makers became increasingly involved in public health, but their attempts to intervene in food hygiene tended to end in failure – for example, in chapter 2 we discussed Edwina Currie's

---

**Box 5.5   Inquiries into the high-status core of the NHS:
Bristol Royal Infirmary (BRI Inquiry 2001)
and Alder Hey Children's Hospital (House of
Commons 2001)**

Context   Bristol Royal Infirmary and the Royal Liverpool
Children's Hospital (Alder Hey) are both high-prestige teaching
hospitals. At Bristol Royal Infirmary, a specialist cardiothoracic
unit provided surgery for children from South-West England
and South Wales who needed complex heart surgery. There
were serious concerns, both inside the NHS and outside, about
the standards of service provided by this unit. Inside the NHS
a whistle-blower, Consultant anaesthetist Stephen Bolsin, called
for an investigation, making his views known not only locally
but also nationally. Outside, rumours started appearing in the
media, e.g. *Private Eye* in 1992, and parents began organising and
campaigning.

   In January 1995, the death of Joshua Loveday on the operating table was the catalyst for an external review. Following this
review, the cases of the unit's two cardiac surgeons and the hospital
Chief Executive were referred to the doctors' regulatory body, the
General Medical Council (GMC), and in 1998 they were found
guilty of professional misconduct. At the same time, parents of
the children who had been operated on in the unit met for mutual
support, formed a group, and in June 1996 called for a public
inquiry. Following the election of a Labour Government in May
1997, the new Labour Secretary of State, Frank Dobson, was
sympathetic to public concerns about the NHS and in June 1998
agreed to appoint an Inquiry into the Bristol service.

   During the Inquiry, one of the medical witnesses indicated
that, without the knowledge and consent of parents, organs had
been removed from babies and children who had died during
surgery and that most of these organs were stored at Alder Hey
Hospital, Liverpool. Several parents wrote to the Secretary of
State expressing their concerns and he responded, indicating that
he would ensure the practice would stop. In December 1999 the
Government announced an Inquiry into the removal, retention
and disposal of human organs and tissue at Alder Hey.

The Inquiries   The Bristol Inquiry concluded that a club culture
in the hospital enabled incompetent surgeons to continue their

harmful practice. The Alder Hey Inquiry concluded the medical profession had concealed from parents the widespread practice of retaining organs and tissue.

The policy implication of the Inquiries Both Inquiries criticised the paternalism of the medical profession and its failure to keep parents fully informed. They provided evidence of the ways in which doctors in prestigious hospitals had abused their position and misused their clinical judgement. They stimulated the shift from professional self-regulation of clinical practice to external scrutiny and regulation through clinical and research governance.

attempt in 1988 to draw public attention to the Salmonella contamination of egg production. The BSE disaster marked a major change (see box 5.1). The BSE Inquiry (2001) exposed a major example of club government, in which those who were responsible for ensuring public safety placed their mutual relations and interests before their duty to the public (Moran 2003: 149). The Inquiry led to a new regulatory regime designed to 'protect public health from risks which may arise in connection with the consumption of food' (Food Standards Agency cited in Moran 2003: 149). One unforeseen consequence of the BSE Inquiry was the extension of the scope of inquiries from disasters that *have* happened to disasters that *might* happen. In the case of mobile phone masts, Burgess (2004) noted that there was no scientific evidence that they caused harm, yet the UK government set up an inquiry into them. In the aftermath of the BSE Inquiry, the Government wanted to regain public confidence by showing a willingness to take seriously and investigate public fears and anxieties about hypothetical risks.

The increasing impact of inquiries

Since the late 1980s the impact of inquiries has increased through the:

- *Routinisation of inquiries* The Government has responded to evidence of repeated failures in high-risk services such as mental health and child protection by creating a system of routine inquiries. Following the publication in 1994 of the Inquiry into the killing of Jonathan Zito, the Department of Health issued guidance to the

NHS that local agencies should set up an inquiry 'independent of the providers involved' (Department of Health 1994: 11) whenever a person who had been in receipt of mental health services killed another person. In 2005 the Department of Health reissued the guidance and extended it to all 'adverse events' in mental health services, for example suicides (Department of Health 2005a). Inquiries were to apply root-cause analysis to identify why the event had occurred and should focus on openness, learning and creating change (Department of Health 2005a: 3). From 1995 onwards, there were on average over fifty homicides a year in which the courts accepted a plea of diminished responsibility (Szmukler 2000: 1) and fifteen published reports a year (Munro 2005). The formalisation of homicide inquiries was part of the overall process of systematising the investigation of 'serious service failures or major dysfunctions' (Department of Health 2001a: 25).

- *Increasing provision of information* We noted above that in 1969, in the case of the Ely Report, the Secretary of State had the final decision over where and how the Report was published. Recent Inquiry teams not only decide what and when to publish but in the case of the larger inquiries, set up their own websites and post interim and final reports, plus all of the supporting evidence. Thus the Bristol Royal Infirmary website includes all the Reports plus full supporting evidence, including witness statements and transcripts of oral evidence (BRII 2001). NHS London has posted all the published independent inquiries into mental health homicides in London on its website (National Health Service London 2010a). Such detailed evidence can be used both for academic analysis of the inquiry process (see, for example, Kewell 2006) and for detailed media coverage of the disasters.

A combination of political and social processes has meant that increasingly in health and social care private misfortunes are treated as public disasters:

- *Development of a risk culture* In chapter 8 we will show that risk has become one of the major ideologies of health care. Judges in the 1980s, such as Lord Denning, argued that the provision of health care was intrinsically dangerous, for example in *Whitehouse v. Jordan and another* he argued that 'Being born is dangerous for the baby' (Court of Appeal 1980: 4), and therefore when a child is seriously harmed or dies during birth that in itself is not 'evidence of negligence'. The Bristol Royal Infirmary Inquiry also noted that 'Heart surgery at any age is a risky enterprise. In babies only months old, surgical techniques are at the frontiers of skill and care' (Bristol Royal Infirmary Inquiry 2001: para3). However, it concluded that, through a statistical analysis of evidence, it could identify preventable deaths (Spiegelhalter et al. 2000). There was a shift to a more litigious blaming culture through the growth of specialist 'no win – no fee' law firms and through increased public funding legal aid. The Department of Health (2001a: 49) estimated that the overall cost of negligence litigation was some £400 million a year with 50 per cent of the bill coming from claims relating to brain-damaged babies. At the same time, the Public Interest Disclosure Act (1998) provided a degree of legal protection for whistle-blowers.

- *Health policy in the policy spotlight* In 1988 the Thatcher review of the NHS intensified the spotlight, with the Secretary of State for Health (Kenneth Clarke), supported by the Department of Health. The post-1997 Labour Government invested massively in health and social care and was committed to modernisation – challenging the powerful provider interests, particularly the medical profession and social workers. Just as Richard Crossman had found the Ely Report helpful in 1969 in his attempts to innovate, so the Labour health ministers found the Bristol Royal Infirmary, Alder Hey and Victoria Climbié Inquiry reports helpful in justifying their programme of modernisation.
- *A feral media* In the 1970s and 1980s new technologies increased competition within and between media and changed the nature of journalism (see chapter 9 for a fuller discussion). The relatively deferential media of the 1950s were replaced by a press that 'hunts in packs' (Blair 2007: 5) and was constantly on the look-out for government error and failure. Thus the media have played a key role in converting private misfortune into public disasters – amplifying risks and shortcomings (Pidgeon, Kasperson and Slovic 2003).
- *Action groups and the public* There has been a continued expansion of pressure groups, and disasters have stimulated the formation of such interest groups. For example, following the killing of Jonathan Zito and the publication of the Inquiry into his killing (Ritchie Inquiry 1994), the Zito Trust (2009) was established to campaign for reform in policy and law. Some groups have played a key role in identifying disasters and calling for inquiries. Parents affected by the Bristol Royal Infirmary and Alder Hey Hospital disasters formed action groups: the Bristol Children Action Group and 'Parents who Inter Their Young Twice' (PITY II). In the late 1990s

the Labour Party was sympathetic and supported the campaigns of such action groups. The public were also given a major role in identifying and reporting problems (Department of Health 2001a: 27). Patients and members of the public could report their concerns not only to local managers but directly to national bodies such as the Healthcare Commission.

Comment

Disasters have had a major impact on policy making in the UK. A disaster is evidence of failure in policy and if ministers are to avoid the blame for the disaster they should immediately sympathise with the victims and take quick and decisive action. They can buy time by appointing an independent inquiry to investigate, but such an inquiry not only indicates the failure of routine policy making but may allocate blame to core policy makers and make recommendations that are uncongenial to ministers. Disasters reduce the scope for rational instrumental policy making: there is little time for cool dispassionate reflection on alternatives when there is pressure to make quick decisions in a highly charged atmosphere. Inquiries do provide a rational response to disasters but it is the rationality of retrospection, when events are viewed with the benefit of hindsight and with an overview that did not exist at the time of the disaster. In such contexts, recommendations and policies are made on the basis of very unusual and exceptional events.

KEY POINTS

- The increasing complexity and scope of modern government means that accidents are inevitable.
- Where such accidents involve high levels of harm and/or are perceived as shocking and a threat to the continuation of business as usual, then they are no longer private misfortunes but become public disasters.
- Disasters reduce the scope for rational policy making by focusing attention on the present or immediate past; creating pressure for immediate action; forcing decision makers to act in the media spotlight in an emotionally charged situation; and undermining the public acceptability of policies.
- Disasters signify a major failure in government policy and policy making which requires special investigation. Inquiries are designed

to restore confidence in government. One way of doing this is to exploit the authority, expertise and trustworthiness of independent experts, especially judges.

- The overt purpose of inquiries is to find the truth. Through the application of hindsight they are expected to identify what happened and why it happened and recommend ways in which such disasters can be prevented from happening again.
- Inquiries also serve more covert purposes, such as emotional catharsis and blame allocation.
- In the early phase of the NHS (1948–68) disasters and inquiries were relatively rare. In this period the mechanisms that could convert private misfortunes into public disasters were underdeveloped. The NHS was protected by the courts. Health policy tended to be seen mainly in terms of providing administrative support. Both the media and the public tended to be deferential and unwilling to raise issues.
- From 1968 to 1988 disasters and inquiries gained prominence, especially in areas that were marginal and peripheral to the main services – long-stay hospital and child protection services. The increasing importance of disasters and associated inquiries was related to major changes in the policy-making environment. The protection of the NHS and related services was diminishing. Health and social care policy making and services moved towards the centre of the political stage. Both the mass media and the public were becoming less deferential and more willing to criticise.
- In the most recent period disasters and inquiries have become commonplace, even routinised, and have been evident in the high-tech centres of medical excellence and in public health. This reflects the reduction in the barriers to identifying problems, for example protection for whistle-blowers and improved mechanisms for identifying and reporting failings, as well as the willingness of Ministers to use the evidence from inquiries to justify modernisation of health and social care services.

PART 2
The Limits of Rationality in Policy Making

6

Identifying policy problems: competition and claims-making

AIMS

To examine the constructed nature of policy making – that the problems policy makers tackle, and the 'solutions' they develop, are decisively shaped by their depiction by a range of interest groups which seek to influence policy.

OBJECTIVES

- To consider a range of different interests which seek to exert influence on policy making and to note the variation in their proximity to power
- To contest rational models of policy making and the way particular 'problems' are taken for granted
- To explore the utility of claims-making models in analysing how problems are constructed, brought to the attention of policy makers, and typified in certain ways
- To understand the ramifications this has for which 'problems' are tackled, and in what way, given the multiple interests which often exist in a particular policy domain.

In the first part of this book we have focused on rational policy making by exploring the ways in which core policy makers – ministers and their advisers – seek to create a better future for citizens. We noted that, in their search for better knowledge, these core policy makers involve others in the policy process. We also noted in chapter 5 that unforeseen events such as disasters could reduce the scope for action to the extent that Ministers invoked the external authority of inquiries to investigate and make recommendations. In the second part of this book we shift the focus of attention to the broader social context of policy making, considering the influence of groups and processes outside the rational inner core of policy making. We start in this chapter with a discussion of the role of interest groups, and particularly their role in identifying policy issues or problems through making claims about the nature of social problems and the best way of dealing with them.

6.1 Seeking influence: insiders and outsiders

Interest groups exist largely to influence both policy makers and the media, often targeting the latter as a route to influencing the former. The choice of whether the media are harnessed in attempting to influence policy decisions, rather than a more direct approach, will often depend on the characteristics of the interest group and particularly its status. Hence the most typical manner of categorising interest groups is as insider or outsider groups. In chapter 4 we described the ways in which insider groups are automatically consulted by policy makers, and those groups whose response policy makers cannot disregard. Within the domain of health policy, the most apparent insider groups have traditionally been the professional organisations – particularly the Royal Colleges, which we discuss in box 6.2, and the British Medical Association (BMA). While concerns over patient trust in the medical professions have been used to limit professional power, especially in terms of self-regulation – discussed in box 6.1 – these organisations nonetheless remain influential within policy-making circles due to their vast levels of expertise.

Policy makers possess very limited knowledge of any one field. Ministers work in one government department for relatively short periods of time and, equally, the tradition of the British civil service has been one which esteems generalised administrative proficiency rather than expertise in any one area (Northcote and Trevelyan 1854). Thus, expertise is a precious commodity and those who can provide it gain increased access into policy making as a result (see chapters 2 and 4). This is especially true in terms of the NHS, in which exceedingly specialised medical knowledge needs to be combined with the organisational–bureaucratic proficiency to run a vast, national institution. Though recent reforms have sought to limit the ability of the medical profession to self-regulate, the form of direct

Box 6.1   Changes to the regulation of doctors

Context   The case of GP Harold Shipman was one of a number of scandals to affect the NHS in the mid- to late-1990s. Whilst the Bristol Royal Infirmary crisis had created concerns that some doctors were practising medicine in a negligent or overly risky manner, the Shipman trial and subsequent public Inquiry dealt with deliberate, gross misconduct in the form of the murder of over 200 patients.

Claims-making   The media coverage of the police investigation, the conviction in 2000 and the public Inquiry which started in September of the same year called for a means of averting a repeat of such a betrayal of trust. The Inquiry in particular was deeply critical of the GMC, which was responsible for the regulation and licensing of doctors. The Chair of the Inquiry concluded that 'the GMC perpetuated a culture of "mutual self interest" among doctors' (Dyer 2005: 10) and recommended that significant changes ought to be made to the way medical professionals are regulated. This added further impetus to the claims made by the Bristol Inquiry, as outlined by Alaszewski (2002).

Policy response   The policy response to such claims has essentially been two-fold – on the one hand, changes to the nature of self-regulation via the GMC have been instituted towards making it more publicly accountable, accessible and transparent; on the other, a secondary system of regulation has been put in place. In this new environment, professional self-regulation is subordinated to the overarching regulatory system of clinical governance to ensure public confidence in 'the standard and conduct of health professionals' (National Health Service Executive 1999: 2–3).

Outcomes   The efficacy of both changes has been called into question. In terms of revalidation, which is a central feature of reforms to the GMC: 'Harold Shipman would, of course, have passed any appraisal of fitness to practise with flying colours. Many of his patients, despite all evidence to the contrary, remained desperately loyal to "Dr Fred," believing that he was the best doctor in the area' (Osborne and Osborne 2005: 546). Clinical governance has also been questioned in terms of its ability to furnish trust (Brown 2008a) and whether it has significant meaningful impact on professional practice (Brown 2008b). Both changes to regulation might better be described as rhetorically useful yet substantively less than effective.

Box 6.2   The influence of the Royal Colleges

Context   There are several Royal Colleges in the UK representing a number of different medical specialities, such as the Royal Colleges of: Physicians; Psychiatrists; General Practitioners; Anaesthetists; and Obstetricians and Gynaecologists. Medical professionals do not have to be members of the colleges in order to practice, although their progression to higher-level posts is usually dependent on them passing the relevant college's exams for membership and/or fellowship.

Claims-making   In contrast to the British Medical Association which specifically represents the interests of its professional members, the colleges' role is more one of furthering and disseminating expertise in their particular field. For example, the Royal College of Physicians perceives its role as aiming to 'ensure high quality care for patients by promoting the highest standards of medical practice. It provides and sets standards in clinical practice and education and training, conducts assessments and examinations, quality assures external audit programmes, supports doctors in their practice of medicine, and advises the Government, public and the profession on health care issues' (Royal College of Physicians 2008: 1).

Outcomes   As a result of their patient-interest basis and unsurpassed level of expertise, the Royal Colleges have a significant level of automatic in-put into health policy decision making as well as 'veto power' (see later section) on training policies.

---

regulation that has replaced this has, through the standard-setting components of clinical governance, granted the Royal Colleges further in-put into how standards are set and the orientation of National Service Frameworks.

The increased importance given to consumers of health care (see chapter 7) has meant that these groups might also be increasingly gaining insider status where policy makers, at a national and local level, seek to include the views of service-users when designing policy. Many of these carer and service-user groups are themselves seen as possessing a certain level of expertise, especially in areas where these interest groups not only lobby but also provide services. Hence Age UK (formerly Age Concern and Help the Aged) is included in certain discussions relating to the provision of health and social care for older people due to its specific expertise and experience of providing services.

In contrast outsider groups are not granted automatic access to the policy-making process. This is not necessarily due to a lack of expertise in the policy area, as a particular group lobbying in one specific area is likely to possess a certain degree of knowledge. Outsider groups lack the status which elicits automatic consultation. They have to use other means to influence the policy-making process. Thus the types of groups which fall into this outsider category may often include promotional groups and those representing economic interests. Promotional groups, or cause groups, are those which pursue an agenda not directly linked to their own interests. Not being either professionals or patients, they do not have a direct personal stake in the NHS, are not consulted due to their lack of explicit expertise in health care, but nonetheless seek to influence policy due to the importance they attach to a particular issue or policy area. In box 6.3 we identify the various groups who seek to influence mental health policy. One of these, the Zito Trust (2009), was concerned with lobbying for mental health policy that counteracts the risk posed to the public by some people experiencing severe mental illness. The Patron of the Trust, Jayne Zito, was the wife of Jonathan Zito who was killed by Christopher Clunis, diagnosed with paranoid schizophrenia, on an underground station platform in 1992 (see chapter 5). Hence, although not directly representing service-users or mental health professionals, the Zito Trust sought to influence policy through raising public awareness of the failings of mental health services and associated policy.

Sectional or economic interest groups are the other main type of outsider group and exist to further their own interests – though, as we noted in chapter 4, during the 'corporatist' period before 1979 some were treated as insider groups. Some organisations representing professionals might also come under this category, particularly the BMA, which is effectively the trade union for doctors and has seen its influence diminished. Outsider sectional groups tend to be businesses which have a vested interest in the way the NHS is run. The biggest of these in terms of both financial worth and public profile

Box 6.3   Interest groups and mental health policy

Context   There are a vast number of interest groups operating in the policy domain of mental health. The Mental Health Alliance, an umbrella organisation under which a diverse range of groups sought to influence proposed changes to the 1983 Mental Health Act (see box 6.5), involved seventy-five different organisations, and yet more exist outside this grouping.

Claims-making   As with many fields within health care, interest groups relating to mental health are of varying types and sizes, and possess varying degrees of influence. Of the insider groups, the Royal College of Psychiatrists is the most established and arguably the most influential. Mind is a long-established interest group which also provides a number of services for those experiencing mental health problems. Both of these organisations can be seen as having relatively similar stances in terms of campaigning for improved quality of services, for equal rights and against stigma.

Perspectives can and do change over time, and the Royal College of Psychiatrists opposed the introduction of Community Treatment Orders – by which patients were to be compelled to receive treatment in the community (Brown 2006). It was actually the College who originally proposed such an idea in the mid-1980s, albeit in a somewhat different guise.

Similarly, SANE (originally Schizophrenia a National Emergency) now explains one of its primary goals as 'to raise awareness and respect for people with mental illness and their families and secure better services' (SANE 2008: 1), whilst in 1988 it used as part of an advertising campaign the following slogans, which were criticised as highly stigmatising: 'He thinks he's Jesus, you think he's a killer, they think he's fine'; 'He hears voices, you hear lies, they hear nothing'; 'She thinks you want to kill her, you think she wants to kill you, they think she'll go away' (see Barnes 1992: 11).

are the pharmaceutical companies. Clearly for these businesses the NHS is a highly lucrative customer. The NHS spends over £7 billion per year on pharmaceuticals – 80 per cent on branded drugs under patent (House of Commons Health Committee 2005: 3). Box 6.4 is a case study of the influence of pharmaceuticals in the case of Beta interferon. A Parliamentary investigation into the effects of the pharmaceutical industry on the NHS suggests this influence is insidious,

---

**Box 6.4   Pharmaceutical companies and their influence –
Beta interferon**

Context   Of all the interest groups which seek to influence health
policy, it is the pharmaceutical companies which are arguably
viewed with the most suspicion. In the UK, where public advertising of prescription medication is illegal, there have been a number
of other means by which pharmaceuticals have sought to boost
sales. These range from lobbying NICE and the Department of
Health, and taking NICE to court over its decision that certain
drugs are not cost-effective for the NHS (e.g. donepezil – see box
7.4), to hosting lunches for medical professionals, and an increasingly close relationship between certain companies and patient
organisations (Herxheimer 2003).

Claims-making   An example of such an alliance between drug
companies and patient organisations involved the prescribing of
Beta interferon for a form of multiple sclerosis. NICE made an
initial decision in 2000 that it was not advocating the use of the
drug. Before this decision had been officially announced, it had
been leaked to the BBC and elicited strong criticism from the MS
Society, pharmaceutical companies and Consultant neurologists.
This sparked a protracted period during which NICE undertook
further research.

Outcome   Just as NICE was about to make public its final
decision, the Government announced that the pharmaceutical
companies would lower the cost of the drug in cases where the
cost-effectiveness of the drug was less evident. This deal between
the Government and the industry undermined NICE's decision
not to recommend the drug, and indicated that 'If the government
had indeed been prepared to incur the displeasure of the pharmaceutical industry when it announced its original plans for NICE in
1997, then by late 2001 there had been a clear retreat from this
commitment' (Crinson 2004: 40).

---

pervasive and, at times, underhand. This influence is held to extend
to society more widely:

What has been described as the 'medicalisation' of society – the belief
that every problem requires medical treatment – may also be attributed

in part to the activities of the pharmaceutical industry. While the pharmaceutical industry cannot be blamed for creating unhealthy reliance
on, and over-use of, medicines, it has certainly exacerbated it. There
has been a trend towards categorising more and more individuals as
'abnormal' or in need of drug treatment, (House of Commons Health
Committee 2005: 4)

This effect is more apparent in the sphere of psychiatric medicine
than elsewhere: 'Psychiatry provides fertile ground for pharmaceutical industry profits because it provides opportunities for
expanding definitions of sickness to include more and more areas
of social and personal difficulty' (Moncrieff 2003: 1). Moncrieff
underlines the ways in which the industry can direct the agenda
for research and its influence over dissemination of findings, and
argues that this calls into question the scientific objectivity of
trials into the efficacy and safety of the industry's products (see
also Smith 2005). Yet the financial power of the global pharmaceutical companies renders their influence extremely difficult
to curb. Their successful ability to lobby the Department of
Health, especially indirectly through the Pharmaceutical Industry
Competitiveness Taskforce, suggests they may be very much an
insider group (Abraham 2009).

6.2 Claims-making as an analytical tool in policy formation

Policy outcomes result from a coincidence of three key elements: a
perception of a social problem accompanied by the availability of
appropriate policy and conducive political circumstances in which
such a policy can be introduced (Kingdon 1995). Whilst interest
groups may propose certain policy solutions, their primary aim is
typically to heighten perceptions of a particular problem. Conducive
political circumstances are out of their immediate control although
if there is sufficient public concern about a particular social problem
then political discussions around this issue are likely to result. Hence
by studying the role of interest groups, it is possible to acquire a
deeper understanding of 'how issues come to be issues in the first
place' (Kingdon 1995: 1).

In developing such an analysis, a model of claims-making is especially effective in understanding the role of interest groups in shaping
policy. A study of claims-making focuses on the social construction
of problems and identifies the individuals and groups involved in this

Identifying policy problems

construction. In this sense, problems do not merely exist – rather, they are constructed by claims-makers who 'try to convince audience members both that a social problem is at hand and that something must [and can] be done to resolve it' (Best and Loseke 2003: 143).

The basis of this approach is a critique of aetiological or realist understandings of social problems. Aetiology is the study of the root of an issue and seeks the solution to a particular problem by offering an understanding of its origin. Yet this model is of limited explanatory value as the roots of social conditions are as multifarious as the natures of the phenomena themselves and aetiology offers no specific framework in order to identify all such causes. In contrast, constructionism is very useful in explaining the problematisation of a wide range of social conditions in that 'by focusing on claims making, constructionists draw attention to something all social problems have in common' (Best 1995: 7). At the risk of being somewhat schematic, there are (at least) four main features common to social problems and hidden within objectivist accounts (see Spector and Kitsuse 1987 for an in-depth account): the arbitrary choice of social problems, the role of claims-makers, the importance of the media, and the power of language in typifying issues.

The arbitrary choice of social problems

Realist accounts portray problems as self-evident, existing independently of the policy process and somehow waiting to be 'found'. There is no questioning of why one issue might constitute a problem and not another, as if the emergence of a social problem were unquestionable. It has been noted already that there are an unlimited number of social issues which could be seen as problematic, yet comparatively few become political problems and develop into the concern of policy makers. The selection process of these problems is difficult to explain in rational terms based on the importance of, or benefits from, dealing with a specific issue as opposed to any other. Rather, claims-makers successfully but arbitrarily attract attention to a particular issue. Such processes display certain compatibilities with incrementalist models (see section 6.3). Rather than the most pressing and serious problems being dealt with, in order of priority, policy prioritisation instead 'takes the form of fragmented or greatly decentralised political decision making in which the various somewhat autonomous participants [in this case decision makers and claims-makers] mutually affect one another, with the result that policy making displays certain characteristics. One is that policies are

resultants of the mutual adjustment; they are better described as happening than decided upon' (Lindblom, 1979: 522).

This 'happening' is evident in the recent history of public and
governmental approaches to the potential danger of violence from
those experiencing mental illness or disorder (see box 6.5). Although
'there was little fluctuation in numbers of people with a mental illness
committing criminal homicide over the 38 years studied [1957–95],
and a 3 per cent annual decline in their contribution to the official
statistics' (Taylor and Gunn, 1999: 9), public perceptions have vac-
illated widely over the same period, culminating in a 'moral panic'
(Szmukler and Holloway 2001: 3) in the early 1990s. This elevation
of the issue at various times, both in the public imagination and in the
priorities of governments which passed, amongst other legislation,
the Mental Health Act (1995) and amendments to the 1983 Mental
Health Act (2007), seems scarcely linked to the generally static
numbers of incidences of violence, but rather a process by which
the issue's 'extent and significance has been exaggerated (a) in itself
(compared with more reliable, valid and objective sources) and/or
(b) compared with other, more serious problems' (Cohen 2002: viii).

The 'reality' of an issue is less important than its *depiction* or representation. Thus policy responses, far from being purely rational and
objective, include distinctly subjective components and 'since society
exists as both objective and subjective reality, any adequate theoretical understanding of it must comprehend both these aspects' (Berger
and Luckmann 1966: 174).

The role of claims-makers

As the use of the term suggests, without the maker, there would be
no claim and hence, though there would exist a number of social
conditions which could be viewed from certain angles as problematic, no social problems would be brought to the public's awareness.
As Berger and Luckmann noted: 'Subjective reality is thus always
dependent upon specific plausibility structures, that is, the specific
social base and social processes required for its maintenance' (Berger
and Luckmann 1966: 174).

In distinguishing between objective reality and subjective construct, claims-making leaves itself open to the philosophical critique
of 'ontological gerrymandering' (Woolgar and Pawluch 1985).
Critics of the approach hold that the distinction between 'reality'
and 'presentation of reality' is in itself arbitrary, as if there were a
clearly definable line between what exists and what is subjectively

**Box 6.5   Reforming the 1983 Mental Health Act –
conflicting claims, muddled policy**

Context   The first step taken by the Government in their attempt to
re-write the 1983 Mental Health Act was to appoint, in late 1998,
an Expert Committee headed by Professor Geneva Richardson to
independently assess the requirements and possibilities for a new
Act. The Committee described itself as having conducted a 'root
and branch review' (Department of Health 1999b: 143), though,
as Lindblom points out, 'this would of course require a prodigious
inquiry into values held by society and an equally prodigious set
of calculations on how much of each value is equal to how much
of each other value' (Lindblom 1959: 79). In spite of this purport-
edly rational approach, the Government then proceeded to ignore
many of the Richardson Committee's suggestions and published
a White Paper, *Reforming The Mental Health Act* (Department of
Health 2000c). The Government's proposals were widely criticised for being coercive, particularly in that they sought to remove
the treatability criterion – a safeguard that ensured that patients
were detained for treatment.

Claimsmaking
Claim A: People experiencing mental illness pose a great risk to
the public and more action needs to be taken to minimise this risk.
    Claims-makers: The government, Zito Trust, most of the mass
media – especially tabloid press.
    Use of media: Highlighting of public inquiries investigating
homicides committed by previous in-patients. More general stereotyping of mental illness (see Philo, McLaughlin and Henderson
1996).
    Typification: randomness and disproportionality, stigma and
otherness. 'I'll sweep psychos off the street: Dobson to cage time-
bomb fiends' (*Sun*, July 1998).

Claim B: People experiencing mental illness are no riskier than
the public at large. They are a vulnerable group of people who
have rights to access high-quality care.
    Claims-makers: Mental Health Alliance – including the Royal
College of Psychiatrists, Mind, etc., professional media and certain
broadsheets – e.g. *Independent*, *Guardian* and *Telegraph*.

Use of media: limited access to mass media (e.g. broadsheets), but the influence of the RCPsych in particular has been significant – arguably as a veto player.

Typification: emphasising the victims of stigma, coercion and poor treatment: 'Mind believes that the provisions for treatment in the community are inappropriate and undesirable. They will not only add little therapeutic benefit, but are liable to backfire' (Mind 2004: 1).

Outcome   In 2006 the Government established a Parliamentary Joint Committee (of MPs and Lords) whose findings were highly critical of the Government's 'fundamentally flawed' proposals. Following this, a Mental Health Act (2007) was passed with the Government having to make substantial alterations to its original proposals and seemingly heed a number of aspects of Claim B.

constructed. These *strict constructionists* would not seek to draw such a line, but would rather hold that, for example, crime statistics or data pertaining to the prevalence of obesity are as much constructs as the claims which are made about them. In this sense, strict construction-ism is 'not concerned whether or not the imputed condition exists' (Spector and Kitsuse 1987: 76) but merely with the way the condition is perceived.

Yet whilst such a position is philosophically more defensible, it is highly limited in terms of policy analysis as it is lacking a framework by which the constructed element of a problem may be separated from the condition itself and thus the ability to elucidate whether a particular claim is reasonable or not. *Contextual constructionists* would argue conversely, that 'audiences and analysts require knowledge of situations and contexts to decode the literal meaning of what they hear or read' (Best 1995: 314). By positing such a methodology within a wider critical realist epistemology, whose theory of explana-tory critique 'opens up the exciting possibility that we may be able to *discover* values, where beliefs prove to be *incompatible* with their own true explanation' (Archer 1998: xviii), the criticism of strict constructionists can be effectively challenged. Certain assumptions with regard to reality are unavoidable (Gordon 1993). Contextual constructionism, however, accepts this inevitability and 'sacrifices analytic purity for sociological knowledge that might help people understand and improve the world' (Holstein and Miller 1993: 244).

It is on this theoretical basis that the role of claims-makers is seen to be vital. It becomes clear that policy makers' foci are often based less on the reality and seriousness of a social condition and more on the successful way in which such an issue has been projected into the public domain: 'The mass public's attention to government issues tracks rather closely on media coverage of those issues' (Kingdon 1995: 57). The success of any claim is dependent on the effectiveness of claims-makers in accessing the mass media. Claims-makers who are more powerful, wealthy and/or media-savvy (in terms of their strategic use of media coverage to further their interests) will therefore find easier access to such coverage and elevate their claim to prominence. This means that the likelihood of a particular issue acquiring problem status is attached to the resources of interests promoting it.

The importance of the media

So far, the media have been depicted as a vehicle used by claims-makers to access the public consciousness, and consequently the attention of policy makers. However, the media are not merely a passive conduit but may act as important agenda setters and claims-makers in their own right (see chapter 9). In this sense circumstances may occur outside the control or planning of interest groups but which elicit attention by their own apparent newsworthiness. This is especially true in disasters (see chapter 5). Outbreaks of the 'super-bug' MRSA in a number of NHS hospitals were reported in the British media from the late 1990s, especially in the run up to the 2005 general election (see Washer and Joffe 2006). These incidents were deemed highly salient for reporting (see box 6.6), without any pressure group working to augment their relevance. Similarly, in terms of mental health policy, one of the most influential incidents was the murder of Jonathan Zito by Christopher Clunis (Laurance 2003). No claims-maker was required to elevate the status of such an occurrence; the media themselves were responsible for the massive publicity the event received and the moral panic that ensued.

Yet whether the media are seen as agenda setters in their own right, or as vehicles for claims-makers to utilise, their influence and centrality in the elevation of certain conditions to social problems and moral panics are beyond question. It is this ability to determine the issues the public is concerned about, as well as to affect *what* they think about these issues, which is the reason why media coverage is so critical to the success of a claim. Media depictions of social conditions have a tendency to homogenise and stereotype (Pickering 2001) in a manner which is exceedingly effectual over

---

Box 6.6   Media as claims-maker – 'superbugs': from MRSA to *C. diff*

Context   Headlines such as 'Danger from MRSA bugs supersedes bio-terrorism' (*Scotsman* 2007) were responsible for a moral panic around the danger of being an in-patient in NHS hospitals. No pressure groups were required to elevate the story to the attention of the media – rather, an exaggerated portrayal in which a patient was more likely to die from a bug than from their reason for hospital admission garnered great media interest.

Process   Whilst MRSA (an antibiotic-resistant strain of a common bacteria) is far from novel (it has been noted since the 1960s), media coverage highlighting the number of wards being closed from infections led to heightened concerns over patient safety and initiated a policy response. UNISON, the public-sector workers' unions claimed that the issue was not so much one of doctors' and nurses' hand-washing but rather that large numbers of hospital cleaners had been cut as a result of the contracting-out of cleaning services over the last twenty years. Ignoring such claims, perhaps due to cost, a campaign promoting hand-washing with alcohol aimed at doctors and nurses was introduced in order to minimise MRSA.

Outcome   Seemingly associated with the imposition of alcohol-based hand-washing, another form of bacteria commonly referred to as *C. diff* (*Clostridium difficile*), whose spores are resistant to alcohol gel, became apparent within a small number of hospitals, leading to renewed media-driven fears over patient safety.

---

public conceptions of certain issues. Moreover, these depictions tend towards representing small numbers of incidents as the norm, thus distorting the proportionality of public views and therefore the reactions of policy makers (Cohen 2002). In this sense, Best notes the paradox that:

> although we consider homicide to be especially terrible, the most serious crime, most homicides are products of mundane motives; they aren't all that newsworthy and they don't get that much press coverage. In contrast, the press is drawn to the most bizarre, the most pointless killings. Reporters rush to tell these stories, but then convert them into representative instances of contemporary violence. (Best 1999: 17)

The media have also played an important role in the construction of mental illness as a threat. Taylor and Gunn's (1999) analysis of homicides showed that people diagnosed as mentally ill made a small and declining contribution to the overall total of homicides. But such an understanding of the condition was absent from the mass media's reportage, apart from in the *Independent* and the *Guardian* (Ferriman 2000). News coverage of statistics and contextualising the small number of such murders within the hundreds of other murders and thousands of road traffic accidents does not sell and does not provoke reaction: 'We do not fear "crime" . . . We fear sudden unexpected, undeserved chaos, pointless suffering at the hands of brutal barbarians . . . this fear of random violence shapes many of our reactions to contemporary social life' (Best 1999: xii). Such media coverage was vital to the formation of a more coercive policy designed to minimise the risk posed to the public by people experiencing mental illness (Pilgrim 2007).

Similarly, the introduction of clinical governance and a wider programme of modernisation was initiated as a reaction to the representation of recurrent failings and negligence across the NHS. The successful way a small number of relatively isolated cases were manipulated to construct an exaggerated fear of the possibility of widespread clinical malpractice was crucial. The crisis thus 'was used by the incoming Labour Government as evidence of the failure of public services and justification of its programme of modernization' (Alaszewski 2002: 375).

The power of language and typification

We noted above the ways in which media reporting can influence the public's understanding of certain social conditions through stigmatising certain groups or through making unusual events appear typical. The ways in which the media use language to describe events and individuals and the links they create between events shape the ways in which problems are highlighted in the media and in the minds of the wider public. As Berger and Luckmann have indicated 'Language is capable of "making present" a variety of objects that are spatially, temporally and socially absent from the "here and now"' (Berger and Luckmann 1966: 174). Claims-makers can use language to conceptualise a condition therapeutically or in terms of fear (Furedi 2002, 2004) in order to engage successfully with media, public and politicians.

Any social condition can be depicted and understood in a host of different ways. The manner in which claims-makers and the media choose to problematise a particular issue will have important implications for the method through which policy makers seek to deal with this concern. Social conditions are never simply 'presented', they are characterised as being problematic in a particular sense. Hence Best (1995) observes how 'typification can take many forms. One of the most common forms is to give an orientation toward a problem, arguing that a problem is best understood from a particular perspective. Thus, claimsmakers assert that X is really a _____ (moral, medical, criminal, political, etc.) problem' (p.8).

As was noted earlier in the chapter, there has been a trend in wider society towards typifying a number of social conditions as medical issues. 'Medicalising' a certain condition tends to add credibility to the claim and therefore facilitates this claim in becoming more powerful and 'real' (Furedi 2004). Referring to a person as *clinically* depressed appears more compelling and serious than simply referring to depression itself. Labelling difficult children as suffering Attention Deficit Hyperactivity Disorder (ADHD) lends greater credence to parents' claims for dispensatory attitudes. Such medicalising claims are, moreover, used by interest groups in the public sphere. For example, war has been recently typified as problematic due to the post-traumatic effects on a country's own soldiers, or meat consumption is negatively portrayed by animal rights groups in terms of adverse mental health effects on abattoir workers (Best 1995; Furedi 2004).

6.3 The predominance of claims expressed in terms of risk

Risk has recently become an increasingly common way of framing and understanding various conditions in health care (see chapter 8). Kemshall has suggested that the concept of risk, 'particularly an individualised and responsibilised risk, is replacing need as the core principle of social policy formation and welfare delivery' (2002: 1). Hence the ability of claims-makers to present their claims in terms of risk is likely to increase the chances of their claims affecting policy outcomes. Late-modern society has seemingly become both increasingly sensitive to the existence of risks and progressively more risk-averse (Furedi 2002). Expressing claims in a language of risk is therefore proving common due to the ability of these claims to draw on such public receptiveness. Moreover, this language is also useful in conforming to the Government's own understanding of many policy issues, as well as performing a legitimising function – claiming validity through 'moral neutrality, objectivity and scientific rationalism' (Jones 2001: 77).

Framing issues in risk-averse ways and using this apparent universal morality as the basis for policy (Furedi 2005: 137) have become highly influential in political debate. Proposals based on such premises appear indisputable. As a result, health-care debates are dominated by risk issues while a number of other concerns, such as the interests of certain, vulnerable groups, remain marginalised (Jayasuriya 2001). Risks to patients or the public are influential in the reputational risk they pose to the Government (Power 2004) and hence claims-makers who, in making their claim, are able to highlight risks posed towards certain individuals or the wider public are more often effective in stimulating responses from policy makers. As we have noted, in recent times health policy makers have been forced to respond to claims about preventable harm in order to allay claims that they do not care and associated reputational risk. Such claims have included that they have failed to minimise the risk of mortality posed by aggressive breast cancer by limiting the use of Herceptin, to prevent violent attacks by a small number of individuals experiencing severe mental illness or disorder, or to identify and take action against 'dangerous' clinicians. The success of such claims has overridden any concerns about the shift of limited resources away from marginalised services to pay for Herceptin, the coercion of vulnerable people experiencing mental illness, or the deprofessionalisation of doctors. Thus the success of claims articulated within a paradigm of risk has led to the discussions surrounding these issues becoming 'disembedded from the politics of power and interests and situated within the *anti-political* framework of security and risk' (Jayasuriya 2001: 1).

6.4 The influence of multiple interests: mutual adjustment and veto players

Opposing claims: Lindblom's model of partisan mutual adjustment

As much as claims expressed in a language of risk may be highly effective, to the extent that the interests of certain groups become marginalised and depoliticised, Lindblom points to the likelihood that 'each value neglected by one policy-making agency [is] a major concern of at least one other agency . . . every important interest or value has its watchdog . . . [and therefore] it can be argued that our system often can assure a more comprehensive regard for values of the whole society' (1959: 85).

Such is the proliferation of interest groups that there are inevitably opposing lobbyists who champion the cause of those marginalised by the claims of other groups. Hence policy makers must not only deal with a multitude of claims seeking to highlight different conditions, but equally try to reconcile an array of competing claims about any one issue. The balancing act of trying to satisfy a number of different claims-makers, and the wider groups in society they represent, is an important part of the democratic process. Yet resolutions between different claims are often problematic due to the highly antipathetic stances of these claims, and their corresponding mutual exclusivity.

In an ideal situation, policy makers would be able to acknowledge all such claims, assess their validity based on perfect information about the conditions they refer to, and come to a rational decision based on such a 'root and branch' review. However, this 'is of course impossible. It assumes intellectual capacities and sources of information that men simply do not possess' (Lindblom 1959: 79). Lindblom goes on to assert that instead of a rational balancing of competing interests, policy making is more accurately viewed as an imperfect amalgamation, or *fudge*, of irreconcilable views. Policy-making is best regarded therefore as disjointed and incrementalist, with the outcomes of this process being highly 'muddled'. For the adjustment between claims does not consider each according to merit but instead is asymmetric, partly determined by the ability of certain claims to capture the public imagination, as mentioned above, but moreover through the compatibility of certain claims with the prevailing ideology of the government (see chapter 8). Thus the 'lopsidedness' of this pluralism actually makes partisan mutual adjustment a far from perfect system of claims arbitration, due to the way that certain important values are inevitably neglected (Lindblom 1959: 81). The unsatisfactory nature of the outcomes for one or more sides creates a tendency for policy makers' rhetoric surrounding a particular policy to become somewhat divorced from the substance of their decisions – as they seek to appease those whose interests have been neglected. Thus the negative outcomes are masked and the whole process becomes further convoluted and distanced from rational, open discussion.

Interest groups as veto players

Such a gap between substance and rhetoric is visible in the various attempts by the Government to revise the 1983 Mental Health Act

(Brown 2006). Early drafts of the proposals 'might be characterized as the iron hand of coercion fitted with the velvet glove of legalism and expressed in a rhetoric of care' (Szmukler and Holloway 2001: 14), yet whilst the 2004 Draft Bill purported to contain 'significant improvements' (Department of Health 2004a: 3), there were few substantive differences from the previous Bill. Difficulties surrounding legislative modification in this area related to 'a structure of veto powers that makes even incremental moves difficult and insufficiently frequent' (Lindblom 1979: 523).

'Veto players are individual or collective actors whose agreement is necessary for a change of the *status quo*' (Tsebelis 2002: 19) and whilst the UK is usually thought of as having just one (Parliament), and therefore the agenda-setting significance of Government is high, there are other organisations within the health-care domain which can be viewed as possessing the veto power to which Lindblom refers. This power lies most prominently with the Royal Colleges, whose status and expertise render any serious objection to a policy difficult to disregard. Ultimately this veto power lies in their representation of the professionals required to implement policy, or carry out new guidelines, thus it is important that a certain degree of consensus is generated.

The failure of policy makers to win over the Royal College of Psychiatrists was crucial in explaining the prolonged delays in replacing, or at least updating, the 1983 Act. The Royal College is an 'insider' group yet distanced itself from the Government's risk-focused stance on mental health (Brown 2006). Normally the asymmetric adjustment between claims would mean that the typification of the problem in terms of risk to the public would have succeeded, in terms both of its use of the media to furnish a moral panic and of the support for this claim by the Government. However, the Royal College can be seen as acting as a veto player and its sustained opposition as part of the Mental Health Alliance, combined with that of a joint committee of peers and MPs who held the 2004 Bill to be 'fundamentally flawed' (Lord Carlile of Berriew, cited in BBC 2005: 1), led to the proposals being significantly changed before being ratified as the 2007 Mental Health Act.

This final outcome in recent mental health legislation perfectly illustrates and substantiates Lindblom's assertion that policy making is a disjointed and incremental process (1959 and 1979). The Government's initial aim of comprehensively reviewing and replacing the 1983 Act was reduced, following much mutual adjustment, to mere modification. The role played by claims-makers on both sides highlights the limitations of more rational depictions of policy making set out in earlier chapters of this book.

Comment

The rational model of policy making starts from the identification of a particular problem or issue. The actual way in which this problem is identified is rarely considered. We have argued in this chapter that 'problems' do not just exist, they are actively created or constructed by claims-makers to shape and structure policy making in their interest. Since there are multiple competing interest groups, there are multiple possible problems and the resources which competing groups can use, such as legitimacy, support and media access, influence which claims are heard. While policy makers may be more receptive to some claims, they will disregard others at their peril if important parts of the media, powerful interest groups and/or the public at large accept them.

KEY POINTS

- The approach of claims-making identifies assumptions latent within objective, aetiological accounts and illuminates the ways in which claims-makers construct social problems.
- As much as political problems may be based very much on constructions, policy makers are nonetheless compelled to deal with them. In certain circumstances this is because they are equally blind to these constructions. Yet even where there is a recognition of the contestable nature of the problem, as long as the wider public perceives a condition as problematic, then politicians are often compelled to react.
- Interest groups not only seek to highlight the existence of a problem but furthermore typify it in a certain light. This often influences the basis on which a potential policy solution is sought.
- As Lindblom (1979) has demonstrated, policies are worked out through a complex causal web of circumstances, conflicting interests and bargaining rather than based on logical resolutions by Ministers and/or civil servants.
- The tension between competing claims forms a more accurate starting point for policy analysis. The power, financial resources and media-savviness of key claims-makers plays an important part in the often lopsided 'bargaining' which occurs around policy

and which typically makes for a rather asymmetrical process of 'mutual' adjustment.

- Amidst these biases towards certain interests rather than others, there may well be a significant gap between rhetorical discussions and substantive changes, thus further distorting the nature of concessions and realignment.
- It is important to note that policy pronouncements are just as much constructed entities as the claims which influence them. From a methodological point of view, this underlines the salience of a constructionist approach for effective policy analysis.
- Objectivist understandings which take political problems and policy responses at face value may be analytically neat, but they offer simplistic and idealised perspectives of the policy-making process.

7

How does the nature of modern democracy shape the formation of health policy?

AIMS

To illuminate a range of influences stemming from the nature of modern democracy that interfere with and obstruct ostensibly 'rational' policy making.

OBJECTIVES

- To examine the ways in which political/civic culture and the electoral system affect both the process and substance of policy decisions
- To emphasise that policy is not made within a vacuum but rather is the product of an array of influences and pragmatic reactions within political systems
- To consider the nature of a 'democratic deficit' and the viability of including patient/public voices in local policy planning.

In the first part of this book we explored the conventional presentation of policy making as a rational process, where expertise is aggregated amidst policy communities and decisions duly made so as to obtain optimum health-care outcomes. However, there are a range of influences on the policy-making process that interfere with and obstruct this ostensibly rational practice. Policy-makers do not operate within a vacuum and thus any accurate analysis of policy formation must account for the range of institutional, social and political-economic factors that influence decision making. In this chapter, we focus on the political context of health policy making and particularly on the ways in which the nature of modern democracy in the UK influences health policy outcomes.

7.1 The nature and influence of democracy

The NHS is inescapably a product of the British political landscape that saw its creation and continues to bear upon it. On a more fundamental level, that the UK is a democracy has important implications for the manner in which health care is managed.

The accountability is in the detail

One function of any effective political system is to confer authority on those who exercise power. This authority is typically based on a combination of rational-legal, traditional norms and/or charismatic characteristics (Weber 1968). These facets are all apparent within the UK parliamentary system. The long history of its institutions and organic constitution offer a traditional authority to those in office that less embedded, more recent democracies lack (see chapter 1). The very presence of this constitution, adherence to it, and the way the Prime Minister and government are elected confer rational-legal authority. The need for party leaders to possess charisma and to harness the media (see chapter 9) would seem to be more important than ever due to the move towards a more 'presidential' political culture (Allen 2003) – one where votes are increasingly won and lost by leaders' rhetorical skills and personalities rather than party policy.

The use of charisma to secure authority and the way this is articulated to the populace via the mass media therefore impose certain limitations on what policy makers can discuss in public. As Rousseau observed: 'wise men, if they try to speak their language to the common herd instead of its own, cannot possibly make themselves understood. There are a thousand kinds of ideas which it is impossible to translate into popular language. Conceptions that are too general and objects that are too remote are equally out of its range' (2008 [1762]: 46).

In this sense, it is conceivable to suggest that, rather than having to 'dumb down' policy discussions to appease the lay-voter, policy making might be more effective if the 'wise man' was given the authority to govern in the interests of everyone, yet without having to consistently justify this to the 'common herd'. Plato (2003) argued that certain people are naturally 'fitted' for leadership and that the masses should leave the job of policy decisions to these experts. It is a very recent phenomenon that mass populations have had any official influence on policy making. And whilst history is littered with accounts of selfish despots, there are also a number of benevolent dictators who arguably ruled in the best interests of the people. Frederick II of Prussia is one example of such a 'philosopher king' (Schieder 2000) in the way that he was (by certain accounts) a highly virtuous ruler: 'clear-sighted, sober, swift, and accurate in his judgements, prompt and unerring in his deeds, an inspired man of action' (Hegemann 1929: viii).

Such a positive appraisal of a democratically elected government would be hard to find. *Clear-sighted* decision making is highly constrained by the multiple interests that have to be regarded in a pluralist democracy. Moreover, *swift and accurate* policies are made less likely by the requirement of being answerable to an adversarial Parliament and critical media. The need to secure legitimacy and thus popularity amongst the 'common herd', and the over-simplification and skewing of policy making that this entails, could be said to make for poorer government. The process of legitimation in an authoritarian state on the other hand minimises the onus on the legislator to present policies which are *popular* and rather enables a focus on maximising the good-life for its citizens.

Singapore is a one-party-dominated state (Jesudason 1999) which has been criticised for its paucity of open democratic credentials, yet one which is economically and socially successful:

> Consider this statement from Lee Kuan Yew, Minister Mentor of Singapore: 'Anybody can join the PAP (People's Action Party) and change the policy from within. If you've got a better idea, you come in, you convince us, you take over' (*Time*, December 12, 2005) . . . One could argue if Singapore had a free press and if its people enjoyed freedom of speech, but one could equally argue that such a regime is feasible [and] desirable. (Ho 2006: 3).

Notions of popularity and legitimacy function very differently in a multi-party democracy. The existence of a free, openly critical media in democratic polities means that policy makers have to prove and justify the feasibility and effectiveness of their policies. In dictatorial or one-party systems, the lack of meaningful elections in which the electorate can eject policy makers from power means there is less pressure on policy makers to ensure their policies are popular, as the threshold for revolutionary action to overthrow a regime, especially a highly authoritarian one, is far higher than the action required to vote a democratically elected executive out of office. Policy-makers within a democracy are generally subject to much higher levels of scrutiny in terms of individual policies and therefore that these policies are amenable to being seen as feasible, legitimate and popular is paramount (Hall et al. 1975). The tension must be noted though between the over-simplification of issues to which Rousseau refers on the one hand, and the increased level of interference engendered by an accountable democracy on the other. The combined effect of these two processes is therefore likely to have a negative impact on the overall quality of policy developed within this system.

The nature and influence of modern, British democracy

There is something particular to *modern* democracy in the way policies are subjected to scrutiny. The gradual extension of the electoral franchise in the UK through the nineteenth century, more or less completed in 1928, was responsible for a change in the nature of representative democracy. No longer able to be known amongst a relatively small circle of their voting constituents, MPs increasingly allied themselves through political parties. This not only enabled more effective exercise of voting power within Parliament but moreover became a way of identifying policy interests and goals to voters. The emergence of clear party ideologies (see chapter 8) through the work of Victorian political leaders such as Peel and Disraeli was accompanied, in line with the gradual extension of the franchise, with the development of mass parties which sought to foster visibility and support in local constituencies.

As the size of the electorate increased, so did the dependence of MPs on parties to win votes. This enabled the parties to exert great influence on MPs voting in Parliament through instructions or 'whips'. Such party discipline, combined with Britain's first-past-the-post electoral system – which amplifies small differences in total votes cast into large differences in proportion of MPs elected, typically resulting in one party with a Parliamentary majority even if it did not attract the majority of the overall vote – means policy making can be a comparatively swift process. The need to build consensus with MPs or other parties is by-passed and hence policy decisions are concentrated within the hands of government Ministers and, moreover, the Prime Minister. Following a close run in the 1988 general election and continued crisis within health-care provision, the Prime Minister, Margaret Thatcher, decided to restructure the

NHS. Within a year she had completed her review, and legislation followed a year later (see box 7.1). Similarly, within seven months of the Labour Party's succession to government in May 1997, *The New NHS: Modern, Dependable* (Department of Health 1997), largely written by one Minister (Alan Milburn) initiated 'the most profound changes ever in the structure of the NHS' (Baker 2000: 16).

Yet the speed by which policies can be enacted in the UK, facilitated by the mass-party and first-past-the-post systems, is counterpoised by both the almost immediate critique affected by the mass media and the straightforwardness of removing parties from power. With regard to the latter, electoral systems would seem to have a bearing on the time-frame within which policy makers operate. For instance, the Swedish Social Democrats have been in coalition government for most of the past seventy years, thus enabling a sustained, consistent development of welfare institutions and policy. In contrast, although British governments have a more absolute ability to enact policy, without the policy bargaining and consensus-building which is typical of more proportionally elected (coalition) governments, there is nonetheless the threat that, if policies are not immediately seen to be effective, then complete removal from government will follow. Thus, whilst Swedish and British models of welfare provision can both be described as having experienced regime change in the past two decades (Pontusson 1997), the NHS seems to be subject to a greater degree of policy tinkering (Klein 1998) than its Swedish counterpart, resulting from the pressure on UK Ministers to demonstrate quick results.

The adversarial nature of the two-party political system is important. Whereas policy makers in coalition governments seek to generate consensus, their single-party-government counterparts have to answer their critics and deflect blame. Clinical governance (see box 7.2 and chapter 1) can be seen both as a response by an incoming government to its criticisms of the former administration whilst in opposition, and equally as a means of altering the system of accountability (Department of Health 1997), and therefore blame (Douglas 1992), within the NHS. By making local service providers 'accountable for continuously improving the quality of their services and safeguarding high standards of care' (Department of Health 1999c: 4), the Government helped to insulate itself from the reputational risk (Power 2004) posed by inevitable failures in NHS services.

The influence of the media has grown since the development of mass democracy required a means by which policy aims and ideologies could be disseminated to a widening audience. Yet the use of the

Box 7.1   *Working for Patients* (Department of Health 1989) – the product of a highly centralised policy-making system

Context   In 1988 the NHS was under increasing financial strain, with real spending having increased by a third over the preceding decade and the Chancellor Nigel Lawson suggesting that further spending rises would not be forthcoming unless the NHS was reformed. Significant change was thus deemed necessary, yet profound changes to the nature of the NHS were politically risky.

Process   Following a high-profile television interview in which Prime Minister Margaret Thatcher committed to review and reform the NHS, and building on an earlier review by David Willets from the right-wing Centre for Policy Studies, a Cabinet team met to review NHS policy and develop a way forward. The general public, MPs and even the medical profession were excluded from this process.

Policy outcome   The highly centralised nature of UK political decision making enabled a radical reform of the NHS to take place within several months, and a new policy document – *Working for Patients* – to be unveiled within a year of the initial BBC *Panorama* interview. The White Paper led to the creation of an internal market, where money was to be distributed to local purchasers (for example fund-holding GPs) who bought services for patients – though health care remained free at the point of access.

Democratic input   The speed of reform and lack of consensus-building says much about the 'elective dictatorship' (Hailsham 1976) of Westminster politics. In stark contrast to the recent protracted bargaining process necessary for President Obama to enact health reform in the US, the NHS review of 1988 was carried out on the terms dictated by the Prime Minister. The concentration of power in the Cabinet ensured that the internal market proposals were merely 'rubber-stamped' by Parliament. That the reforms were heralded through a television interview demonstrates the media-driven authority of the Prime Minister.

Box 7.2   Alan Milburn and *The New NHS: Modern, Dependable* (Department of Health 1997)

Context   In 1997 the newly elected Labour Government was keen to make their mark on the NHS – the most prominent feature of the welfare state to which the Party had traditionally been so committed. Yet, while in opposition, the Chancellor-to-be, Gordon Brown, had committed the Government to keeping within Conservative budgetary forecasts for public spending at least for the first year.

Democratic pressures   On the one hand, a new policy was required to make evident to the electorate that 'New Labour' were committed to change – 'we will be the party of welfare reform', promised Blair (cited in Powell 2000: 39) – while on the other, the policy had to be cheap. Any large-scale investment or building programme was out of the question in the short term.

Personality   Alan Milburn was a young, talented, imaginative junior minister within the Department of Health. He can be described as a policy entrepreneur (Rose 1996) as opposed to other ministers who may have had less opportunity and/or decisiveness and imagination to impose their own political will. *The New NHS: Modern, Dependable* 'had a much stronger input than usual from Ministers and particularly the Minister of State, Alan Milburn (it is rumoured that the final version of *The New NHS* was completed on Mr Milburn's laptop computer)' (Baker 2000: 8).

Process   Manifesto promises such as cutting waiting lists by 100,000 in the first year were shelved, and the absence of a dynamic Secretary of State at the time created an opportunity for Milburn. The highly centralised nature of the British system, combined with the vast majority enjoyed by Labour in Parliament at the time, meant that the new policy was able to be instituted more or less immediately.

Outcome   One individual Minister was able to have a significant impact on the running of the NHS due to a range of contextual and personal features as well as the nature of the British parliamentary system. The policy of clinical governance (see box 1.8), first set out in *The New NHS*, was heralded as 'by far the most ambitious quality initiative that will ever have been implemented in the NHS' (Scally and Donaldson 1998: 61).

media by politicians to publicise policy plans and accomplishments is double-edged – the media can be critical of policies. We shall explore the influence of media upon policy making in more detail in chapter 9, but here we should note that the media are utterly central to the nature of the modern democratic process, shaping public beliefs about, and confidence in, the government and the political system. While the media can provide rational critiques of policies based on reasoned discussion of the limitations of policy approaches, policy makers are concerned that they create fictitious constructions of social problems or policy failings for which little evidence exists. The Department of Health has called for responsible media in the following way: 'The media also have a responsibility to ensure that a proper and legitimate role in revealing problems and holding services to account is balanced with the need to avoid the level of sensationalism and distortion of the facts which will lead their readers, viewers and listeners unjustifiably to lose confidence in the NHS as an institution' (Department of Health 2001b: 8). The 'sensationalism and distortion' referred to above, not to mention the 'reality' of policy errors, have come to be seen as such a risk to the political capital of governments that ministers have increasingly sought to 'manage' the media coverage of the executive, and thus the risk posed to their reputation. This resort to 'spin' (see chapter 9) leads to a policy-making process which comes to be driven more by the manner in which policies are presented than by the efficacy of their implementation on the ground.

Habermas (1989) bemoans the loss of an era in the nineteenth century when a small, bourgeois public sphere facilitated undistorted communication and the exercise of public reason. In this period, the role of the press was simply to 'mediate the reasoning process of the private people who had come together in public' (Habermas 1989: 188), and therefore policies and ideologies were articulated, debated and critiqued in a relatively thorough, undistorted fashion. In this setting, 'public opinion' was the product of this public exercise of critical reason – offering emancipatory potential as part of an Enlightenment project. But as the media increasingly became a market-driven commodity, 'public opinion was no longer a source of critical judgement, but became a social-psychological variable to be manipulated' (Scambler 2001: 4).

It is within this context that the inherent irrationality of policy making begins to emerge. The democratic process, now a mass procedure, is unavoidably reliant on a media which, in their modern guise at least, distract from reality and reason, to the extent that policy making is no longer able to be grounded in either. Therefore, when returning to Hall and colleagues' model of effective policy (1975), the consequent manner in which feasibility, legitimacy and popularity function is made highly problematic. Feasibility comes to be understood in an increasingly short-term way, in which the sacrifice of instant goals for long-term gain, or difficulties in the embedding process of new policies, are unacceptable amidst a climate of adversarial politics and sensationalised criticism by the media. The development of 'spin' to counteract this distorted scrutiny leads to a situation in which the day-to-day feasibility of policies becomes less important than their 'media-appropriateness'. Feasibility is better understood, thus, not so much as the functionality of policies but rather as the way that they are *seen* to be working.

Mass democracy, of course, underlines the importance of policies acquiring popular support, though there would seem to be an increased blurring between what is meant by popular support and legitimacy. If legitimacy is the compatibility of a policy's means and ends with commonly shared beliefs or norms (Parsons 1949), then the late-modern plurality of norms and values induces a more pliable notion of legitimacy which 'is likely to vary with the ideology of the party in power and with its suppositions about what "public opinion" or important interest groups consider the limits of State action to be' (Hall et al. 1975: 476). In this ambiguous normative context, as long as a policy is popular – or at least not highly unpopular – then it is legitimate. The various attempts to redraft the 1983 Mental Health Act between 2000 and 2006 highlight the process by which the support of the general public encouraged 'governments to act in ways which were, in any one case, damaging to the interests of some individuals, groups or classes' (Hall et al. 1975: 483) – in this case, people experiencing mental illness. Whilst, as we noted in chapter 6, the presence of certain interest groups as veto players (Tsebelis 2002) may act to protect the rights of such groups (Lindblom 1959), the blurring of legitimacy with popularity makes this task all the more difficult.

7.2 Involving the public in health policy decisions: democratising or meddling?

The impact of public opinion on health policy is paradoxically both essential and problematic. The manner in which democracy facilitates accountability for individual policies is, unlike in a dictatorship, more likely to ensure that seriously flawed or incompetent policies are illuminated and rectified. Yet the manner in which the media manipulate public opinion may mean that what is depicted as problematic or flawed is not 'objective' but constructed through media representations. Hence, though democracy is perhaps the 'least worst' of all alternatives (Winston Churchill, cited in Rose, Mishler and Haerpfer 1998: ii), it nevertheless may be less effective at making health policy than a benevolent, technocratic dictatorship: not only is public understanding of health care distorted by the media, but it is also highly limited in the first place.

The nature of health-care policy decisions requires exceedingly high levels of expertise – in terms of the application of highly sophisticated sciences of medicine and epidemiology coupled with the organisational complexities of a vast health-care organisation. The lay public possess little understanding of these systems of knowledge and therefore might be said to be ill equipped and under-informed to warrant inclusion in the decision-making process. The basic economic problem of health care, in which rising expectations and complex needs lead to infinite demand for scarce, limited resources, inevitably entails a degree of health-care rationing. Certain services or treatment must be provided at the expense of others. Yet this overarching necessity is difficult to articulate to a general public for whom the notion of health-care decisions being taken on grounds of economic rationalism appears immoral and thus compromises trust: 'most patients are uncomfortable with the idea that their doctor must balance their needs against the needs of others. If patients truly knew the extent of developing conflicts of interest built into existing financial and organizational arrangements their trust would be much diminished' (Mechanic 1995: 1657).

Therefore it is possible to argue that the public not only lack the organisational awareness to make decisions over service provision, but are better served as patients when decision making is limited to the experts. The consequences of excessive public involvement in policy decisions such as rationing, can be seen in the case of Herceptin (see box 7.3).

The campaign to widen and standardise the availability of the drug successfully harnessed media support, and as a result the Government overrode its own directives to Primary Care Trusts in terms of spending constraints and evidence-based medication. While public opinion understandably supported the rights of breast-cancer patients to an apparently highly effective drug, the decision to compel Trusts to provide the drug would unavoidably have required the withdrawal of services in other areas, for which there may well have been a stronger evidence base. In this sense, the 'democratisation'

Box 7.3   Herceptin revisited

In box 2.8 we set out considerations surrounding the prescribing of Herceptin in the NHS from a narrow, rational policy-making perspective. However, when we consider this example within the wider political context of the democratic system, the picture becomes somewhat more complex (see Hedgecoe 2004).

Context   Research trials of the drug Herceptin confirmed its apparent efficacy in reducing mortality rates when targeted at women diagnosed with the aggressive HER2 form of breast cancer. Later data also suggested benefits for early-stage sufferers. At the same time, local Primary Care Trusts (PCTs) were under increased pressure to control their spending in line with centrally imposed budgets, making a number of PCTs reluctant to advocate the prescribing of Herceptin due to its cost.

Process of mediatisation   Supporters of women denied the drug organised campaigns to highlight their cause. Instances such as affected mothers with their young children presenting a petition at 10 Downing Street attracted media attention. Media reports such as the BBC's *Panorama* programme highlighted the apparent 'postcode lottery' whereby certain women living in one area were prescribed the drug whilst others were denied such treatment. Some media accounts obscured that Herceptin was only of significant benefit for HER2 sufferers, that the technicality and further costs of HER2 testing were great, and that the drug had potentially lethal cardiac risks.

Policy outcome   As a result of heightened media pressure, the Prime Minister, Tony Blair, requested a Department of Health directive ensuring that all PCTs allowed the prescription of Herceptin for HER2 patients at early (as well as advanced) stages, undermining the usual delegation/decentralisation of budgetary decisions to local PCTs. As a result, many PCTs had to cut spending on other services.

of health-care decision making may well lead to the tyranny of the 'media savvy' over the marginalised, in which young mothers with aggressive breast cancer are judged more newsworthy than elderly or mental health patients (see boxes 7.3 and 7.4), with the former

Box 7.4   Drugs for treating Alzheimer's Disease which mainly affects older people

In contrast to the successful overriding of a decision on the cost-effectiveness of Herceptin, the prescribing of drugs for early-stage sufferers of Alzheimer's disease, such as donepezil (Aricept), remained unfunded by the NHS over a number of years, following the ruling by NICE (see box 7.7) that the drugs were not cost-effective.

Context   Cost-effectiveness testing of the drugs by NICE was based on tests of cognitive functioning (Mini Mental State Examination, or MMSE) and on this basis NICE only recommended that the drug be prescribed to benefit those with moderately severe Alzheimer's (MMSE score of 10–20).

The campaign   Pharmaceutical companies and carer/patient groups such as the Alzheimer's Society campaigned for those with early stages of the disease to be able to receive treatment. The campaign received a modest level of media attention. NICE maintained that its stance was based on appropriate research which showed negligible effects. Opponents criticised that NICE's decision was based on a narrow conception of patient benefit, such as cognitive function, without taking account of wider issues such as quality of life for carers.

Policy outcomes   In spite of campaigners' attempts to obtain a High Court injunction challenging the decision, the NICE directives continued to advise against the prescription of the drug to early/'mild'-stage patients (though a new appraisal announced just as the book was going to press in 2011 has extended the availability of donepezil and some similar drugs for early-stage Alzheimer's sufferers).

acquiring costly, effective treatments at the expense of the latter, who receive a 'Cinderella service' (Means and Smith 1985; Bernard and Phillips 2000). In box 7.4 we discuss the failure of the campaign to overturn the NICE directive that drugs such as donepezil (Aricept) should not be prescribed for early/'mild'-stage Alzheimer's patients as there was insufficient evidence of cost-effectiveness.

Overcoming the democratic deficit

In spite of the limits of public knowledge and awareness of issues as discussed here, there has been a recent trend in the UK towards increasing public and user involvement in health-care decision making. Baggott (2005) describes how the long-standing, yet largely ineffectual, convention for public involvement at local-level decision making was revitalised through the 'new managerialism' of the early 1990s. Those buying-in or 'commissioning' services within the internal market were encouraged to take into account the concerns of local service-users (National Health Service Management Executive 1992). Yet the continued paucity of public or patient influence was highlighted by the high-profile *Voices Off?* report (Cooper et al. 1995). The proximity of the publishers of this report, The Institute for Public Policy Research, to the incoming Labour administration of 1997 helps explain the latter's interest in expanding and enhancing the means by which public and patients could influence local health-care provision.

This late-twentieth-century concern with a lack of public in-put into policy formation contravenes previous understandings of the role of representative democracy. Unlike the earliest democracy of the Greek city-states in which the minimal number of 'citizens' enabled their direct involvement in policy decisions, democracy in modern nation-states is representative. Edmund Burke's eighteenth-century understanding of this notion saw the representative as elected based on esteem of his character and judgement – thus able to act autonomously after the election under the sole condition that he could be removed at the next election. Burke's own failure to gain re-election after articulating such a conception arguably adds credence to the alternative 'mandate model' in which a representative is elected on the understanding that they will act in keeping with certain assurances about their stance on various policy issues, usually articulated within a manifesto.

The conception of a 'democratic deficit' sees such a model as insufficiently stringent in holding policy makers to account. Since elections occur so seldom, governments, particularly in a highly centralised state such as the UK, are able to function as *elective dictatorships* (Hailsham 1976) once in office. Furthermore the complexity, range and depth of late-modern policy formation entails that the decisions made by policy makers are far too numerous and detailed to be adequately articulated in a manifesto. As Kingdom has argued, 'the powerful few in Britain extended the franchise to the mass, and did so in a way calculated to minimise damage to their own privileges' (Kingdom 1991: 127). Sizeable cuts to public services in the face of widespread opposition, as announced in 2011, would seem to support this assessment – yet the hiatus in health reforms announced by Secretary of State for Health Andrew Lansley also points to the potential for influence between elections (box 7.5).

7.3 From patients to health-care consumers: great expectations

Recent government discussion of overcoming this democratic deficit and including users in decision making is often tied to a conception of these service-users as consumers rather than patients: 'We live in a consumer age. Services have to be tailor-made not mass-produced, geared to the needs of users not the convenience of producers. The NHS has been too slow to change its ways of working to meet modern patient expectations for fast, convenient, 24 hour, personalized care' (Department of Health 2000a: 26). Since the 1980s, the notion of democratic deficit has been focused at the individual level rather than the collective or corporate one (see chapter 4). The golden age of parliamentary democracy, in which reforms were MP-led, had been replaced by the mid twentieth century by a Whitehall club of ministers and civil servants. While this club government began to unravel from the late 1970s, policy making under Thatcher continued to be highly centralised (box 7.1). Post-1997 Labour governments have taken the notion of consumer rights and public in-put more seriously, culminating in *The NHS Plan* (Department of Health 2000a) based on extensive public consultation (see box 4.5).

More than simply the legacy of 'a consumer age', the transition towards health-care consumers can also be seen as a recent outcome of a long transitional process in the way knowledge is managed in health-care interactions between medical professionals and patients (see Alaszewski and Brown 2007). The progression, through informed consent, away from the protective, paternalistic model towards a more involved, less deferential, role of the patient has culminated more recently in a degree of patient choice (see box 7.6). Medical professionals acting as advisers who make patients aware of the potential benefits and risks of a course of treatment, but with the patient making an informed choice, have in this sense replaced the traditional role of the physician as an agent making decisions on the patient's behalf. The new function of the patient as

Box 7.5   The Lansley hiatus

Context   Alongside sweeping reforms and cuts across the public sector, in January 2011 the Coalition Government announced proposals for consortia of GP practices to take over the commissioning and managing of health-care services from Primary Care Trusts. Widespread concern was voiced from across a range of representatives within the medical profession, nursing, the charity sector and a number of patient groups – not least in relation to concerns over the format by which private companies could bid for contracts, as well as representation on consortia boards. This opposition was echoed across the public sphere – from significant numbers signing petitions against the reforms, to media personalities speaking out against the proposals, to musical critiques on YouTube.

Policy of listening   On 4 April 2011, the Government announced that it was going to 'pause' its plans for NHS reform, referring instead to the inauguration of a 'listening exercise' in order for the 'details' of the new policies to be finalised with the in-put of NHS professionals and the public. The outcomes of this exercise were still to be seen when going to press yet there had already been adjustments in policy – for example, away from GP consortia towards 'GP-led' consortia, suggesting the involvement of a wider range of stakeholders in the commissioning bodies.

Direct democracy or a political game?   A two-month pause in policy in the face of public and professional disquiet is quite unprecedented in NHS policy-making processes. The previous Labour administration had made much of its own form of 'focus group' listening approaches but these were pre-planned rather than part of a hiatus following criticism. It remains to be seen how influential this 'listening' is and the extent to which ideology makes this exercise highly selective as to what is 'heard' (see chapter 8). Yet the exercise nonetheless represents a novel departure in quasi-democracy. The coalition format of the Government and the apparent disagreement over health policy between its Liberal Democrat and Conservative members may also be a significant contextual factor which led to the listening exercise. Hence, such a possibility for in-put and dialogue is perhaps more aptly seen as the result of an amalgam of political features, rather than a straightforward reaction to heightened critiques in the public sphere.

Box 7.6   The patient choice agenda

Context   There has been a gradual move away from a paternalistic ('doctor knows best') basis of medicine, through increased provision of information and use of this within consent, towards the current 'patient as consumer' model of health care (Alaszewski and Brown 2007). At the same time, recent health policy since 1997 has been very much preoccupied with the concept of quality and how this can best be elevated at all levels of NHS provision.

Process   While this combination of consumerism and concerns over quality might be seen as logically progressing to an introduction of choice, further impetus was provided by the party political debate in the run-up to the 2005 general election (Appleby and Dixon 2004). Conservative proposals for giving patients the option of a public/private mix of funding procedures may therefore have encouraged the Labour Government to push ahead and further develop plans to guarantee patients' choices between health-care options funded entirely by the NHS. Since the institution of the internal market under a Conservative Government in 1992, means of increasing incentives and levers towards improved performance have been contested. Whilst the more explicit talk of an internal market proved distinctly unpopular due to fears that the market would compromise patient care, 'patient choice' is a more palatable means of ensuring competition within the NHS. Hence choice represents both media-friendly rhetoric and a viable policy solution to the political problem of incentivising quality care. Moreover, favourable political circumstances encouraged the policy onto the Government's agenda.

Policy outcomes   This development, combined with recent policy commitments to high-quality care, has culminated in the institution of a patient choice agenda (Department of Health 2004b, 2006a). Examples of such choice include the 'choose and book' system, by which Consultant appointments can be made instantaneously at the GP surgery. Whilst this may be seen by a number of GPs as putting increased pressure on their short 10-minute appointments, it is a successful means of ensuring patients get an appointment with which they feel satisfied. Further examples of choice include pharmacy provision of repeat prescriptions.

decision maker in their health care has been formalised and extended in recent policy developments to include 'how, when and where they receive treatment' (Department of Health 2006b).

Two assumptions underpin this policy development: first, the assumption that patients have the capacity to make decisions about how, when and where they receive treatment and that such choice is in their long-term interest. The 'adviser model' suggests that the patient will be fully informed of the appropriate details by the appropriate medical practitioner, though whether they are able to take on-board sufficient information to make an effective decision depends on both their own capacity to understand and the communication skills of the professional. Choice is thus not necessarily conducive to improving outcomes, for example for those with chronic conditions where choice may damage continuity of care (Ferlie et al. 2006).

The second assumption is that service-users actually desire choice. Coulter (2005) points out that, whilst there is not unanimous support for choice, particularly with regard to chronic patients, the most important issue for people is the availability of quality services when needed. The danger in terms of encouraging patients to choose between services is that it will be inferred that choice is based on a differentiation in quality between these services. Confidence in the standardised quality of services may therefore be compromised by knowing that some services are better than others.

This deviation in standards is unacceptable in an era of high and ever-rising expectations of health-care provision. The move from deferential patient towards health-care consumer brought with it greater assumptions about the form of service provision the service-user is entitled to. A public appreciation of health care, free at the point of access, apparent after 1948, has been replaced by increasing demands on, and dissatisfaction with, levels of NHS provision: 'Memories of the fragmented and inequitable system that preceded its introduction are fading . . . and the NHS can no longer trade on people's gratitude' (Coulter 2002: 186). Treatment through the NHS is thus seen not so much as a beneficial service but more as a natural right, and consequently limitations of service provision are tolerated less.

Consumerist tendencies in the health-care sector can be traced back to the wider development of consumerism in the 1970s, epitomised by the Consumer Association and its publication *Which?*. The expansion of such provision of public information on commercial goods and services into the public sector, particularly health care, has been endorsed and encouraged by a range of policies visible since the late 1980s. *Working for Patients* (Department of Health 1989) was one of the first White Papers to formally recognise the NHS as structured around the consumer, rather than as essentially a productivist (profession-led) organisation. *The Patient's Charter* (Department of Health 1991b) enshrined such a consumer focus, offering what was effectively a patient's bill of rights, as well as underlining entitlements for recompense in cases where these rights were not upheld.

While the charter ceased to function after 2001, the notions of entitlements are still very much emphasised in later policy documents, with 'choice, responsibility and empowerment' being the essential vocabulary for NHS White Papers (Newman and Vidler 2006). In spite of the limitations of emphasising choice already mentioned, the notion seems to be at the centre of policy thinking, for example through *Building on the Best: Choice, Responsiveness and Equity in the NHS* (Department of Health 2003). Equity as applied in the 'new NHS' takes on a different meaning from its original 1948 usage, when people exercise their choice they are treated differently rather than all the same.

Responsiveness is thus about tailoring health care to individual needs. Though one may question whether in fact these are largely middle-class needs, the responsiveness issue is seemingly driven by the irreconcilability between rising expectations, expensive new treatments and an ageing population, on the one hand, and increasingly constrained resource provision, on the other (Taylor-Gooby 2006). Coulter (2002) describes the problematic paradox in which 'public spending on health care is increasing much faster than inflation in most countries, and effective treatments are available more widely than ever before . . . [yet] at the same time, public pessimism about the future of health systems is growing' (p. 186). Responsiveness is an attempt to deal with the latter, seeking to ensure the increasing resource provision is more effectively applied to best satisfy consumer expectations – countering the deficit of public control. Policy is oriented towards making health care more transparent in order to 'shift the balance of power' (Department of Health 2002) in favour of the consumer, thereby maximising the potential for meeting their expectations. In this sense 'consumerism is likely to form an increasingly important *regime of surveillance* as targets about responsiveness and choice become more centrally embedded in processes of audit and inspection' (Newman and Vidler 2006: 207). Where patients are referring to their own experiences and therefore have much to contribute, a confusion over exactly how to take these opinions into account has seemingly led to an inertia in aggregating such perspectives into decisions over service delivery (Rowe and Shepherd 2002).

Dealing with expectations: a 'new' and accountable NHS

At the beginning of the chapter we noted that the key difference between democracy and its alternatives was the level of accountability those in power were subjected to. In attempting to limit the democratic deficit and manage the expectations of a new generation of 'health consumers', it has also been suggested that policy makers have increasingly tended towards the imposition of accountability frameworks. By making providers accountable for maximising the quality of service provision (Department of Health 1999c: 4) and offering patients a choice between certain of these providers, policy makers have effectively created a quasi-democratic NHS in which patients can *vote* through their *choice* of service provider and treatment.

In the same way that Parliament institutes checks and balances on the Executive through the 'eternal vigilance' (Kingdom 1991: 295) of the committee system and question time, health-care providers have recently been subjected to heightened levels of scrutiny through various systems of monitoring and surveillance, effected through the imposition of targets, protocol and audit. The results of such audits and monitoring are being made more freely available to the general public, with the apparent aim of ensuring that local providers are answerable to their consumers for the services supplied.

The original emphasis of such policy (Department of Health 1997 and 1998b) was the standardisation of service provision across the country, in response to an increasing awareness of the existence of a so-called 'postcode lottery'. Such variations in standards of treatment were highlighted by the Calman and Hine (1995) report which found the form and level of treatment for various types of cancer varied markedly between different hospitals and health authorities. This creates another contradiction, as policy makers are simultaneously seeking to ensure the similarity of service provision through standard-setting and the monitoring of compliance with these benchmarks, while providing consumer choice which will facilitate diversity of health-care experience. In this sense 'we have to understand how consumerism as discourse attempts to link a number of different ideas – about history, about modernity, about equality, about public services – into an uneven, uncomfortable and often contradictory alignment' (Newman and Vidler 2006: 207). A tension thus exists between meeting expectations at the national democratic level (of one NHS for all), and the flexibility required to satisfy local democratic objectives.

Building trust in the NHS: legitimacy chasing its own tail

Such contradictions are apparent in the other key aim of accountability policies – rebuilding trust in the NHS: 'Patients will be guaranteed national standards of excellence so that they can have confidence in the quality of the services they receive' (Department of Health 1997: para . 1.4). At the heart of the accountability framework and assurance of standards is the concept of clinical governance, which in turn is explicitly based around the notion of trust – 'interest in clinical governance has erupted because individual practitioners have betrayed the public's trust' (Maynard 2003: 31). Evidence of such betrayals included the series of 'catastrophic failures in bone tumour diagnosis in Birmingham, paediatric cardiac surgery in Bristol and cervical screening in Kent and Canterbury' (Freedman 2002: 133) which surfaced during the late 1990s (see chapter 5).

The disasters which we discussed in chapter 5, including the removal of organs from deceased child patients without parental consent, which occurred at the Alder Hey hospital in Liverpool, added to this growing list. Bristol in particular has been described as 'a watershed in the development of health and social care services in the UK' (Alaszewski 2002: 371), in that it was seen as illustrating more endemic failings in the system as a whole (Smith 1998). Alaszewski (2002) notes that what set Bristol apart was its status as a highly reputed institution, making the failings all the more shocking, as well as the similarities in the findings of the subsequent public Inquiry to reports into cardiac services at other 'centres of excellence', such as the Royal Brompton, Harefield and Oxford.

Also critical was the level of media coverage Bristol received, and it is arguably this reporting, coupled with heightened attention paid to failings in Birmingham, Kent and Canterbury and others, which brought the issue of clinical quality onto the policy agenda. The successful way the relatively isolated failings were manipulated to construct an exaggerated fear of the possibility of widespread clinical malpractice within the NHS was crucial. In 1997 the incoming Labour Government was able to use this crisis as a tool for building support and perceived legitimacy for its programme of modernisation and governance.

Such machinations have been successful in constructing a crisis of trust in the NHS. For, as much as trust was said to have been irreparably damaged by such incidences, there was little evidence to support this. On the contrary, 'despite Harold Shipman and other high-profile examples of malpractice, the public has clearly decided these are the exceptions which prove the rule; trust in doctors has increased over the past two decades' (MORI 2004: 3). Hood (2005) notes that, even during the specific years of Bristol, Shipman et al., public trust in the medical profession remained steadfastly high.

Hence, the first inconsistency apparent in the introduction of clinical governance is that it has essentially been motivated by a trust crisis which is more apparent in media reporting and policy rhetoric than in public opinion. Furthermore, if there has been a crisis of confidence in the medical profession, the systems of monitoring and surveillance surrounding clinical governance are not necessarily useful in ameliorating such a situation. Hood (2005) describes the contradictory, Orwellian 'doublespeak' that is visible within policy rhetoric, whereby policy makers label NHS agencies Trusts but do not trust them. This lack of faith in service providers and clinicians is demonstrated by the manner in which accountability and organisational controls are evidence-based to the extent that trust is negated (Scambler and Britten 2001).

Thus there is an apparent contradiction between policy rhetoric and outworking: 'Because we trust people on the frontline, the centre will do only what it needs to do . . . The centre will not try and take every last decision' (Department of Health 1997: 6.6). Although a number of decisions are delegated by the centre, the 'performance monitoring' and 'inspection' cited in the previous paragraph underlines what is meant by 'trust', which, rather than possessing any real substance, acts more as a rhetorical 'velvet glove' within which the 'iron fist' (Jermier 1998) of coercive accountability (Shore and Wright 2000) is loosely hidden.

These contradictions may only act to damage public confidence rather than rebuild it. For example, the Department of Health has created a website which 'gives people the opportunity to directly share their experiences and generate user ratings of the services they have received' (Department of Health 2006b: 8). Whilst on the one hand acting as a useful check and balance over service provision, the illumination of variability in experiences is likely to damage the confidence of people accessing such information, particularly if their local organisation is rated negatively. If users see an agency as legitimate when they perceive it as 'just, benevolent, in their best interest, and deserving of their support, loyalty, and adherence' (Frank 2000: 1), recent policy approaches could be understood as being based on the notion that the NHS has been suffering a legitimacy crisis. Yet by attempting to make the NHS more open, responsive and accountable, policy can be interpreted as promulgating a conception of the medical profession as closed, self-serving and beyond scrutiny. Moreover, the manner in which accountability, monitoring and surveillance frameworks function tends to emphasise the measurable at the expense of the more 'human' elements of health care (Harrison and Smith 2004). So attempts to make the NHS more accountable to the public do not necessarily enhance the patient experience.

Though seeking to elevate the concerns of the individual patient and ensure an experience of quality of care, *good practice* is reduced to 'a matter of convention, efficiency and "internal coherence"' (Marcuse 1989: 121) due to a largely numerical and systematic focus of audit and control which tends to concentrate on systems rather than individuals (Power 2003). Hence, instead of being elevated and empowered, the concerns of the individual person may actually become subsumed by targets and protocol. Thus, in the case of legitimacy and trust, 'the government desire for measurement is such an unsatisfactory way of improving public services because what matters is never measurable and what is measurable rarely matters' (Kennedy 2004: 162).

Clinical governance illustrates the contradictions and irrationality which the pursuit of popularity and democratic legitimacy can create. A media construction of a crisis of legitimacy and trust, and concerns over the responsiveness and accountability of the NHS, have actually led to policy which in some senses undermines the concerns of the individual human being receiving treatment and may heighten anxiety about the dependability of the services being provided. This latter issue is further underlined by the creation of the National Institute for Health and Clinical Excellence (NICE) as a key component within the clinical governance framework. NICE (see box 7.7) exists to disseminate protocol and directives based on cutting edge, evidence-based clinical practice research. For example, it makes decisions on drugs to be prescribed in the NHS in order to ensure the standardisation of medication provision. Yet this role has served to publicise the inevitability of rationing that occurs within the NHS, a factor which undermines patient trust (Mechanic 1995).

Clinical governance has greatly accelerated this awareness, and in the process stimulated public anxieties about health-care provision. Making decision-making processes more explicit and visible, rather than leaving them to individual clinicians, would seem to lead to a system that may work more effectively, but in which people trust less – increasing rather than reducing the democratic deficit (Alaszewski and Brown 2007).

Box 7.7   National Institute of Health and Clinical Excellence (NICE)

Context The basic economic problem of any publicly funded institution, not least one where expectations are always rising and the cost and potential for treatment is ever expanding, is one of infinite demand and limited resources. In this context, health-care rationing of some form or other is inevitable. Modes of rationing are visible throughout the NHS in various more or less subtle forms: 'rationing by delay (waiting lists), discrimination (against the elderly and mentally ill), dilution (two nurses on a geriatric ward at night when there should be four), and diversion (long term care moves to the social sector)' (Smith 2000: 1364). Where rationing occurs in an ad hoc, covert form, the potential for inequalities is high.

Policy and debate   NICE was set up as a de facto rationing agency to determine which drugs/treatments were cost-effective and which were not, to develop protocols and guidelines of evidence-based best practice, and, based around this, to generally facilitate quality health-care decisions in the NHS. One of the most contentious issues is that "it's living a double lie" (Smith 2000: 1363). First, it pretends that its primary function is not health-care rationing when this is indeed the case. Second, it presents decisions as to why certain treatments are approved or not as if this was simply a case of sufficient evidence for effectiveness or a lack thereof. The decision is far more political than that. As boxes 7.3 and, particularly, 7.4 highlight, decisions over Alzheimer's patients' pharmacology cannot be reduced to mere scientific rationalism, but rather must inevitably incorporate and be influenced by concepts such as identity and notions surrounding the 'moral meaning of old age' (Gilleard and Higgs 2000: 22).

Comment

There is a case based on the arguments raised in this chapter, for insulating policy decisions from the negative, 'irrationalising' effects of democracy. In the same way that the setting of interest rates has been moved from being a Treasury responsibility to being that of the Bank of England, it would seem that putting health policy decisions in the hands of a small number of expert technocrats may result in a more rational, effectual decision-making process. It would certainly help limit the level of policy tinkering to which the NHS is currently subjected. Yet whilst the setting of interest rates does invariably have a crucial impact on the financial status of the country, and consequently on individual livelihoods, the decisions taken by the Bank of England do not involve directing the way in which £100 billion of tax-payers' money is spent. This matter, combined with the affective, human and moral elements of health care, make it harder to insulate it from the public sphere. Hence, whilst a move towards a more technocratic, depoliticised management of the NHS would make for more 'rational' policy formation, it is precisely the same elements of democracy which encourage irrational policy making that would make such a transfer impossible to enact.

KEY POINTS

- The pursuit of *popular support* in modern democracies may often represent a dysfunctional influence on the rationality of health policy. In order to achieve this support, policy makers must respond to media constructions rather than more rationally conceived, evidence-based problems.
- The adversarial nature of political debate in the UK means that, in order to be seen as *feasible*, policies are designed around ostensible, superficial success in the short term rather than the longer-term effectiveness of the policy.
- What is feasible in terms of the scarce and limited resources of a publicly funded NHS is often irreconcilable with the ever-increasing expectations of health-care consumers.
- Attempts to create a more open, accountable and responsive NHS have led to the compromise of expert decision making, increased bureaucratisation at the expense of the individual, and the publicising of health-care rationing and system failures which may serve to increase, rather than dispel, public anxieties about quality of service delivery.
- Enshrining the rights and increasing the in-put of patients, though limiting concerns over a democratic deficit, also act to encourage the consumerist impulse of patients and public which engenders inflated expectations of health-care provision that are essentially incompatible with the inevitable rationing of a state health-care system.

8
Ideology and policy: legitimating, bounding and framing

AIMS

To explore ideology as a concept, and the ways in which policy makers are embedded within ideologies while also using ideologies to legitimate policy and thus themselves.

OBJECTIVES

- To explore ways in which ideology has been understood as well as noting the lack of agreement over its conceptual limits
- To consider the role of ideology as a tool of legitimation, in linking practical policy decisions with particular commonly held values and norms
- To note the usefulness of ideology in *framing* policy dilemmas, for example as a medical, legal or social problem, which is essential for these to be tackled, thus emphasising the highly constructed nature of policy formation. In this way ideology 'bounds' the rationality of decision making – distinguishing important issues from those which are beyond interest.
- To analyse the development of three significant recent ideologies in health care – risk, choice and regulation – and consider their impact on health-care systems and policy decisions.

In chapter 7 we described the ways in which the nature of liberal democracy structures the formation and implementation of health policy. Central to this structuring is legitimation – through the formulation of policies which are seen to be in line with prevailing societal norms and values (Parsons 1949). But the requirements of popular authority and their influence on 'effective' policy making are far from straightforward, as we will show in this chapter.

8.1 Ideology as a concept – power and what is possible

The sheer breadth and depth of policy concerns (from expansive new programmes to the minutiae of resource allocation) mean that a great deal of policy making is beyond the attention or interest of the voting public. The absence of awareness and in-put that such ambivalence creates means that other mechanisms for steering policy are essential and it is here that ideology plays a key role both in ensuring consistency across, and in providing legitimation for, policies.

It is important that there is consistency amongst the different sources of direction so that policy making, across the vast remit of the welfare state and beyond, is sufficiently 'joined-up'. The complex inter-dependencies and complementarities of diverse policies (for example, the quality of private and public housing stock affects respiratory health) require overarching schemes for routing diffuse projects around one general orientation. Furthermore legitimation within democratic systems is a much broader phenomenon than that pertaining to government (Eagleton 1994) – opposition parties also require means of garnering support and authority (beyond the Weberian notion of charisma seen in the preceding chapter), despite lacking the ability to enact public policy.

Fulfilling these multifarious requirements is the concept of *ideology*. Its versatility and nebulous characteristics make it a problematic notion to 'tie down'. The concept is one that elicits much debate and contestation amongst those writing about it. Gann (1995) draws out many of these characteristics as they appear amongst a number of key texts. In its earlier usage a dualism emerged between ideology as a 'science of ideas', as put forward by the Enlightenment philosopher de Tracy, and Marx's use of ideology as a more insidious notion by which political power over the masses is gained surreptitiously (Eatwell 1993).

The exercise of power is at the centre of many analyses of ideology, not least those following Foucault (see Burchell, Gordon and Miller 1991), and is more explicitly evident through the spectres of totalitarianism – either communist or fascist. The application of *ideology* in these regimes posits it in terms of an all-encompassing doctrine – more political paradigm (or worldview) than discrete policy compass. Associated with this approach are conceptions of ideology as an *insidious deceiver*. This understanding of ideology as influencing society 'behind our backs' is the starting point for the critiques of various social theorists drawing on psychoanalysis – notably Žižek (1989, 1994) – rooted in Lacan, and critical theory (as summarised in Habermas 1987: 380), employing aspects of Freud. Whilst these concerns are beyond the scope of this textbook, essential to both is the level at which ideology functions – more specifically, whether it is an inescapable lens (Eagleton 1994), a 'fantasy' which shapes our reality (Žižek 1989) or a mode of social control which is struggled against.

Such analyses of power, in underlining the role played by ideology in creating assumptions as to what is real, normal or important at the most fundamental of levels, make clear the scope of its influence. For whilst notions of rationality are often employed as self-evident and unquestionable (as seen in the earlier chapters of this book), considerations of ideology make starkly apparent how even the most fundamental orientations of scientific modernism, or capitalist economic growth, have respectively emerged out of the humanism of the Enlightenment (Adorno and Horkheimer 1972) and Calvinist perspectives on redemption (Weber 2002 [1930]).

Therefore the prevailing or accepted 'patterns of ideas' (ideologies) at any one point in time are shaped by that which has gone before – flowing out of, or in reaction to, preceding ideologies, e.g. New Labour's Third Way as a response to Thatcherism which was a reaction to the perceived failures of post-war Keynesianism (see box 8.1 for fuller discussion). They limit the conceptions of what is possible, knowable or 'right' for policy in the future. In other words the function of ideology is to provide a basis for a rationality, creating a paradigm within which policy possibilities can be deemed effective or dysfunctional. As a result of this process, however, ideology also blinkers policy making within highly restrictive bounds of what is feasible, popular and appropriate.

Thus ideology poses at least two significant problems to the rational policy model: where ideology is a tool in political contests (aimed at vote-winning) it has the ability to warp decisions and so 'ideological policy making' and spin preclude or usurp rational, informed debate; where ideology is dominant, embedded and unquestioned, it limits the scope of policy considerations and the rational weighing up of alternatives.

8.2 The utility of ideology for policy making

Legitimation – winning and mobilising popular consensus

Foucault's (1984) conception of ideology provides an insight into power – both the power exercised by producers of knowledge/ideas in promulgating assumptions as to what is 'true' or normatively valid, and the positions of political-economic power which are maintained by this knowledge-hegemony. These considerations may seem rather abstract and distanced from practical policy making in relation to the domain of health, yet will become much more pertinent in a later section when we turn to notions of framing and *spin* – as personified by Alistair Campbell – in influencing and setting the agenda of popular debate in the public sphere.

The association between ideas and power, and how this bears upon legitimacy, is indeed central to much of this chapter. Ideology is uniquely capable of relating commonly held assumptions of what governments should be pursuing with practical policy decisions – thus attaching legitimacy to the latter. Ideological tools, in presenting the linkages between policy options and norms and values, are able to win or dispel support through this association between decisions and that which is normatively appropriate. Over time it is also possible that this ideological dissemination is able to shape or re-characterise assumptions as to what policies are necessary and desirable: *Habeas corpus* (right to trial before incarceration) has long been seen as a basic part of the rule of law on which a healthy society functions (enshrined in the Magna Carta of 1215: Holt 1992). Yet by characterising terrorism as a problem of inadequate security, and by focusing on risk and danger as a grave threat to society, *habeas corpus* has been deprioritised (within recent UK anti-terror legislation) by reconstructing the linkages between policy and values – thus legitimating the control of terrorist suspects without trial.

As the work of Žižek (1989) on ideology, and the experiences of totalitarianism, make evident, it has an intrinsically *utopian* element. It implies there is a 'good place' (which currently does not exist but which could be reached or rediscovered), and a correct path to follow if society is to arrive there. The visions of communism or fascism were explicit in this regard, and more violent in its pursuit – yet *all* ideology, at its core, combines considerations of what is normatively good, correct and desirable, and a methodology of how this end is most effectively pursued in a more practical sense (Eatwell 1993: 13).

The linkages between the conception of a goal and understandings of how this should best be reached were highly visible in the early history of the NHS. An assessment of the inception of the service makes evident the importance of a growing consensus – a collective assumption as to what was normatively valid – around an ideology that a universal health-care system, free at the point of access, was necessary and appropriate for post-war Britain. Another prevailing ideology – that of the supremacy and utility of medical knowledge and the Consultants who embodied this – helps explain why the new organisation of the NHS became run around producers (i.e. doctors) in the way that it did (see also box 4.2).

More recently, the development of a consumer-oriented worldview – that the customer is always right – is an integral piece in the jigsaw of understanding recent reforms within the NHS, not least the advent of 'choice' and competition (see Le Grand 2007). In this sense notions of prevailing patterns of thinking and policy practice are very much bound up with one another (Heywood 2007). Concerns of legitimacy – the need to be 'in-step' with commonly held norms and values (Parsons 1949) – explain this close association. For if decision making deviates too far from normative consensus, then the policies enacted may be unworkable (for example amongst professionals) or the decision maker will lose authority and thus power.

Bounded rationality – problematising issues and claims-reception

By focusing attention on risk and safety, or by harnessing the tool of choice as a locus of health policy, policy makers not only legitimate their authority but, moreover, make the process of decision making less complicated. A further utility of ideology therefore is the way it acts in providing boundaries between that which should be the concern of policy makers and that which is insignificant – narrowing the policy focus to a relatively small number of considerations. This notion of 'bounded rationality' was set out by Herbert Simon (see chapter 3) and can be partly characterised as relating to the benefits of 'docility' (Simon 1982: 202): that decision making benefits from receiving certain ideas via instruction (from socialised norms, or in our case ideology) rather than empirical investigation of every single case or eventuality.

As we discussed in chapter 6, policy makers face not only an infinite number of possible issues they could deal with, and have myriad resources of information at their disposal, but moreover face a vast number of interest groups who seek to influence the decision-making process. The sheer complexity of this would be paralysing were policy makers not to make use of tools for 'muddling through' this quagmire of contingency (Lindblom 1959). To this end, ideology is one effective means of defining what is problematic and the basis by which problems can be solved – therefore precluding a wide number of other concerns from policy consideration.

This role of ideology in giving policy makers predisposed, receptive interests (selective hearing) towards certain issues, which inherently engenders ambivalence towards others, can be understood more precisely through Osborne's notion of problematisation:

> It might, however, be useful to substitute the notion of problematization for that of constructionism. Instead of saying what issues of health policy are simply constructs (constructs of what? Of power?), it can be said that such issues are always the product of particular problematizations (Foucault, 1988). Problematizations are not modes of constructing problems but active ways of positing and experiencing them. It is not that there is nothing 'out there' but constructions but that policy is fundamentally a creative rather than reactive endeavour, it also means that policy can never just be about anything (as often appears to be the case with the more insistent form of constructionism). On the contrary, the function of problematization is to reduce complexity, to provide a field of delimitation regulating what can and cannot be said. (Osborne 1997: 174–5)

This excerpt sheds light on how ideology not only drives what is focused on, but provides the lenses and therefore approaches by which social conditions are perceived and tackled. In this sense the terms 'problematisation' and 'ideology' may be considered as relatively synonymous – with risk, once more, providing a pertinent recent example of a concept which characterises phenomena in a particular light, thus profoundly shaping the format of policy 'solutions' to these conditions.

The process of framing – defining actors and interests

Ideologies, as has been made clear, exist at the nexus between political concepts and practical action. This is not a unidirectional relationship. The Private Finance Initiatives (the co-ordination of private investment to fund public infrastructure) exist as a practical outcome of a prevailing ideology of the Third Way – see box 8.1 – yet considerations in the public sphere of their appropriateness and utility range between 'securing better public services' and 'backdoor privatisation' – themselves ideological positions. This latter process,

> **Box 8.1   The Third Way (see, for example, Giddens 1994)**
>
> Informed by the perceived failure of Keynesian and monetarist economics, and the unpopularity of neo-liberalism and traditional social-democracy, the 'Third Way' was the ideology on which the post-1997 Labour administrations were grounded. A middle road between market liberalism and state interventionism, some key hallmarks of the ideology were:
>
> •   Role of government is to enable, not command, and the power of the market is harnessed to serve the public interest
>
> •   A strong civil society enshrining rights and responsibilities, where the Government is a partner to strong communities
>
> •   A modern Government based on partnership and decentralisation, in which democracy is deepened to suit the modern age.
>
> This public–private hybrid is apparent across a number of health policy initiatives – from Private Finance Initiatives (PFIs), to patient choice, to the public health initiative 'Choosing Health' – in which individuals are deemed responsible for their health (neo-liberalism) but the state intervenes to make healthy choices easier (paternalism).

that of characterising practical policy decisions in specific form, language and rhetoric, makes plain the final function of ideology addressed in this section – the process of framing.

The procedure of framing a policy, or indeed any action or decision, is an intrinsic feature of the social world (Berger and Luckmann 1966) – utterly unavoidable. Each social condition is only understandable by media of communication, whereby every narrative or picture used by an actor to convey a decision has certain associated connotations and values imbued within it. This cultural framing through language – based on common assumptions of the deeper meaning latent within certain words, phrases and concepts – ensures that political, aesthetic and moral sensibilities are inherently raised when any policy issue is discussed. Indeed, the language used inescapably comes to typify the issue. Therefore the stance taken by a pronouncement on a certain condition will greatly affect the size and type of constituency it resonates with, for example in asserting that a certain issue is really a moral, medical or political problem (Best 1995: 8).

As we argued in the discussion of bounded rationality, this form of framing is an important prerequisite of policy making. Framing an issue in a particular light ensures a clarity of focus as regards the key actors, responsibilities and interests involved. Merely considering that obesity is a problem will do little to deal with the issue. Instead, characterising the condition as a result of late-modern society, class, transport or the profligacy of certain diets is the first stage towards tackling the issue and vital in delineating the range of stakeholders who are responsible or who need to be engaged with. Hence framing – as a means of putting ideas into action – is an integral role of ideology, and emphasises the instrumentality of the concept.

Yet this inherent typification carries many dangers with it, such is the power of language in making actors conscious of the world in particular ways, where certain realities are emphasised ahead of others (Berger and Luckmann 1966: 174; see also chapter 6). Framing, in characterising a social condition in one particular light, usually precludes many other salient concerns and therefore makes a more holistic, effectual solution less likely. The medicalisation thesis (e.g. Illich 1976) would contend that by understanding obesity, for example, as a medical problem inevitably blinds policy makers and the public to understandings of the social contexts which drive rising levels across Western societies. Furthermore, there is often a maxim of blame latent within framing, which, at least in the case of obesity, typically points to the flaws of the individual rather than the social and economic features of modern society which structure and confine individual action. Although harnessing medicine and the NHS might, prima facie, appear to be a logical, objective response, critics argue that the growing policy interest in public health is grounded in a neo-liberal absconding of the state's responsibility towards the welfare of its citizens.

8.3 Evolving ideologies and the changing position of government towards health

The past two centuries have seen a perpetual shifting in the ideologies of health and health care, and the responsibility of the state towards these. Such prevailing 'patterns of ideas' exist within medicine, public opinion and policy circles – a trilectic with all three increasingly bearing upon one another. For much of this period, as with preceding times, the role of the state in health and health care was a minimal one. In line with the prevailing liberal (i.e. limited government) ideologies of the 1800s, as espoused by contemporaries of the era such as John Stuart Mill, the power of government was seen as enshrined around individual freedom and rights, only intervening where there was concern over harm to others (Mill 1993).

In this sense policy issues relating to health were acutely bounded by such a framing of the 'good-life' as being brought about by minimal state interference. Any significant expansion of the state's role at this time would have thus been deemed illegitimate, with the state over-stepping its role and engendering tyranny. The first legislation explicitly focused on health was the 1848 Public Health Act. The concerns over harm to the public relating to the availability of good-quality drinking water and effective drainage, as highlighted by Chadwick's Report on the Sanitary Condition of the Labouring Population in 1842 (Baker n.d.), thus made possible this initial incursion of the state into this domain. Where significant mortality (public harm) existed in local areas, local health boards were allowed to be set up and taxes could be levied to pay for improvements to infrastructure.

Although public health issues were in this way established as legitimate territory for state intervention, the general provision of health care (via General Practitioners and hospital medicine) remained quite firmly within the domain of the private and third sectors. Guy's hospital (founded in 1721) was one of many charity foundations providing health care to the urban poor and as the 1800s progressed, local co-operative forms of health insurance were gradually set up by a number of local communities. Prevailing liberal norms and values within British society facilitated state intervention only to the extent of regulation, with the 1858 Medical Act establishing the General Medical Council to assure minimum standards for doctors. Hence in contrast to Bismarck's Germany of the late nineteenth century, which ensured relatively widespread access to health insurance for workers, the provision of health care in the UK was not co-ordinated or assured in any way by the state. Access therefore was typically limited to the rich, elements of the poor and destitute (where local charities or co-operatives existed), and the insane (through asylums – though any notions of 'care' provided here are disputable).

As with the British context, Bismarck's Government was staunchly Conservative in ideology. Its introduction of insurance legislation for health (1883), accidents (1884) and old age / disability (1889) was elicited as a response to the perceived threat from the growing support for another ideology – socialism (Hennock 1998). By bringing in welfare reforms Bismarck was successful in linking his own administration with the concerns of the people – thus heightening his own legitimacy and that of the newly unified Germany, whilst

---

Box 8.2   Ideology as reaction to prevailing ideas and socio-political environment: President Thabo Mbeki and AIDS (1999–2004) (see Paroske 2005)

Mbeki rejected the orthodox view that HIV was causally linked to AIDS and influentially questioned the theory that the illness was spread through sexual contact. In the face of significant criticism for this stance, Mbeki 'made the case that South Africa's unique experiences under apartheid demanded a strong tolerance of dissent and debate' (Paroske 2005: iv). Hence this stance can partly be understood as a reaction against Western-colonial dominance and subjugation of black South Africans. It is also a phenomenon of the specific political and socio-cultural environment of South Africa at the end of the twentieth century.

Problems Widespread impact of disease, dependence on Western pharmaceutical companies, cost of treatments (manufacturers of anti-retrovirals had refused to market drugs at affordable prices for the African market).

Ideology Post-colonialism – need for separation from the dominance of Western political economy.

Policy Support of alternative viewpoint rooted in traditional medicine and southern African cultural approaches to health and illness.

---

undermining the critiques of the left. This policy enactment thus underlines that ideologies never develop within a vacuum, they are inevitably reactionary (Catholic hegemony – Reformation – counter-Reformation; modern capitalism – communism – Solidarity in Poland; Western cultural/political imperialism – radical Islamism); moreover, they are a fusion of already-existing notions within the crucible of particular economic, political and social conditions, as with President Mbeki's response to AIDS, discussed in box 8.2.

The success of a Labour Government in the 1945 UK general election is ideologically complex, yet nonetheless evidence of the ability of a newly popular ideology to harness wider public reactions to quite peculiar social, political and economic conditions in Britain as it emerged out of the 1939–45 war. Ideology serves both to harness support and to orient public opinion in new directions. The success of the 1945 Labour administration in these two domains is made apparent through its initial victory, alongside its enduring legacy. For in spite of losing the 1951 general election, a new post-war consensus had been inaugurated, with Conservative Governments until 1979 accepting the new framing of the state's role (or duty) in providing comprehensive health and social care.

Whereas the liberalism of the 1800s had bounded decision makers away from expansive state intervention, the post-war ideologies of democratic socialism and One Nation Conservatism galvanised assumptions and confidence in the quasi-utopian possibilities of state involvement in many aspects of economic and social life. However, the increasingly globalised forces which had contributed to the conditions by which these ideologies could flourish in the first place (via war and substantial post-war economic growth) similarly acted to undermine these very assumptions and confidence in 'big state' policies. The oil-market-induced price shocks of the 1970s and resulting 'stagflation' (concomitantly high unemployment and inflation) were held by opponents of state interventionism to illuminate the fallacy of the underlying economic ideology (Keynesianism) on which it rested.

As a result, a new set of assumptions – rooted in monetarist economics and neo-liberal political thought – became the new loci for co-ordinating policy decision making. Issues relating to the running of the NHS therefore increasingly came to be framed around the innate inefficiency of the public sector, with responses to these problematisations being bounded or blinkered towards the superiority of private-sector competitiveness and management norms. This starkly redefined the actors and interests of the NHS in the 1980s – with policy advice and direction increasingly being sought from private sector experts (most notably Sir Roy Griffiths, see box 2.4) and the decade culminating in the NHS being enshrined as a consumer-led institution through the Patient's Charter (Department of Health 1991b).

Alongside a more consumer-led approach, the NHS of the 1990s witnessed a reinvigoration of ideologies stressing the responsibility of the state for public health (Department of Health 1992, 1999a). As in the 1800s, these have been said to develop out of fundamentally liberal (albeit now neo-liberal) political assumptions (Petersen 1997): the need to limit the size of the state (i.e. NHS spending) by focusing on individual responsibilities and autonomy. The co-option of the general public in monitoring and assuming responsibility for their own health (and that of their peers) highlights the ideological trilectics referred to at the beginning of this section. The medicalisation of issues such as obesity (see Campos 2004), sexual performance (Tiefer 2006) or happiness (Pilgrim 2008) is shaped by, and in turn shapes, policy and public perceptions of the remit and utility of medicine in late-modern society. The recasting of these conditions as health-related at once invokes stigma around those who fail to look after their health and puts pressure on policy makers to intervene through the NHS.

8.4 Late-modern ideologies and health policy: regulation, risk and choice

Two key themes which serve to tell us much about the nature and functioning of ideology are:

- that ideology gradually evolves – and is a reaction towards previous dominant assumptions. Where these assumptions are explicit and contestable, then 'new' ideologies are able to react against these and distance themselves from their predecessors – in this way creating new assumptions as to the desirability of certain 'ends' and effective 'means' for pursuing these. Where assumptions have become so embedded as to be utterly unquestioned, then the reshaping of ideology is itself bounded/limited by these existing assumptions.
- ideologies exist at many different levels, as is shown in box 8.5 – hence, prevailing ideologies which problematise obesity (as discussed above) are themselves informed by wider assumptions about the role of government and society in the surveillance of public health, which in turn may be seen as flowing out of a more fundamental neo-liberalism (Petersen 1997).

These two themes will become quite evident as we move now to assess more contemporary ideologies and their role in legitimising, framing and bounding health policy decisions.

The evolution of ideology is evident in the development of Labour policy in the latter years of opposition and early years of government from 1997. Commonly referred to as the 'Third Way', this new ideology was a reaction against Conservative tendencies towards more overt forms of marketisation whilst very much constrained by the precepts which, following Thatcherism, had become uncontestable (Heffernan 2000). The 'legacy' of Thatcherism (Heffernan 2000) ensured that any reversion towards more traditional democratic socialism was impossible – instead an often uncomfortable hybrid of neo-liberalism and enhanced regulatory tools (Moran 2003) emerged, described by one more critical commentator as "Thatcherism with a Christian Socialist face" (Jessop 2006: 2).

Informed by the accepted 'failure' of Keynesian economics and traditional interventionist social democracy, yet seeking to earn legitimacy through offering an alternative to the unpopular neo-liberal and monetarist tendencies within 1990s Conservatism, the incoming Labour administration pledged to dismantle the internal market of the NHS, which was portrayed as bureaucratic and compromising quality and safety (Department of Health 1997). That this quasi-market was still an underlying basis of the NHS a decade later (Sheaff and Pilgrim 2006) highlights the gap which often exists between the rhetorical goals of ideology and the substantive policies which do not necessarily follow these. Ideology may therefore be as much about 'rebranding' existing functions as it is about galvanising change.

Labour reforms have thus sought to place concerns over 'quality' at the heart of the NHS, rather than preoccupations with efficiency (Department of Health 1998b). And whilst the substantive actualisation of quality frameworks (through clinical governance) cannot be contested, the continued existence of 'efficiency fetishisms' (Jones 2001) as a component of quality (Brown and Calnan 2010) and the New Public Management drivers behind this framework make clear that the 'New' NHS is very much a legacy of its predecessor's ideological DNA. Indeed, the remaining three themes to be discussed in this chapter – regulation, risk and choice – can each be understood not so much as novel creations but rather as more or less logical continuations of existing policy themes. Each of these progressions, though often framed in quite novel ways, is typically bounded by that which has gone before (Lindblom 1959).

Regulation – enabling rather than commanding?

One hallmark of the 'Third Way' which continues to act as a cornerstone of government policy is the ideology of government as an 'enabling' rather than commanding force, in order that the power of the market is harnessed and regulated to serve the public interest. Here the notion of a middle way between interventionist socialism and free-market neo-liberalism is plain. Policy making is accordingly bounded by notions that, on the one hand, the market is a useful, efficient and preferable means of providing welfare and other services but, on the other, the market needs regulation and governance to prevent failures (due to lack of provision or poor-quality provision – i.e. a lack of signals and incentives).

One example of this 'enabling rather than commanding' hybrid has been the building of NHS hospitals through Private Finance Initiatives (PFIs), a form of Public–Private Partnership (PPP). Whereas the possibility of any private sector involvement in NHS delivery or capacity would have been precluded (or bounded out) by pre-Thatcher ideology, this pragmatic solution to the need for new infrastructure in spite of budgetary limitations fits neatly within the wider, now legitimate, framework in which private-sector investment can be harnessed, regulated and contracted to meet the needs of welfare service delivery (with the added bonus of reduced Treasury interference in infrastructure planning). Hence the initial problema-tisation and framing of the issue of a lack of NHS infrastructure has been oriented by the between-market-and-state ideology of the Labour administration. In turn, these practical manifestations of the overarching ideological position become assumptions in their own right – organising principles of how future investment should be co-ordinated within specific areas of the public sector. The two key themes introduced at the beginning of this section are thus clearly apparent – the gradual progression or evolution of ideologies, and the multiple levels at which ideologies exist: from the more abstract (in-between-the-market-and-the-state) to the more practical (PFI as a common framework to finance NHS capital investment).

This tendency within policy making is characteristic of the wider move away from a confidence in state intervention (see box 8.3), as undermined by the economic conditions of the 1970s, towards a growing confidence in the state in its ability to effectively regu-late a growing number of domains within the public and private spheres. Moran (2003: 155), in describing how a previously stable UK system of governing underwent dramatic and pioneering shifts towards a regulatory state, underlines the significance of a *vision* of 'a rule driven, non-discretionary regime' (2003: 107). This ideology of striving towards the pinnacle of 'good governance' has in turn been driven by assumptions and norms around the importance of 'hyper-innovation; justifying innovation as the search for policy effec-tiveness' (2003: 171).

Ultimately, Moran suggests that the regulatory state emerged out of the ruins of an untenable institutional arrangement of 'club rule'. The 'fiascos' attributed to such discretionary and ad hoc decision making, combined with the perpetual and defensive policy tinkering which an adversarial parliamentary system inculcates (Klein 1998),

---

Box 8.3   From 'big government' to the 'Big Society'

The shift away from command-and-control towards enabling forms of governance is most recently epitomised within the Big Society ideology of the Conservative-led UK administration. The central concern of this approach is 'a massive transfer of power from Whitehall to local communities' (Cabinet Office 2011a) – the premise being that government intervention undermines the social fabric and social capital of communities and that the withdrawal of the state will enable 'civic energy' to flourish (Cabinet Office 2011b).

This vision is criticised from a number of angles – Law (2008) argues that ideologies underlining the significance of 'social capital' can be used as a guise for the abdication of responsibility by the state for social problems and failing communities. Kumlin and Rothstein (2005) meanwhile underline the role of state welfare services in establishing and undergirding social capital. In this sense, a number of the policies which are outlined under the umbrella of the Big Society – not least private contracting of welfare services – can be deemed problematic in the way that they reduce the visibility of the *public* practice of compassion through the welfare state (Brown and Flores 2011).

The wide range of policies bracketed under the Big Society suggests the danger of an ideological concept being stretched so broadly that it loses its clear link between values and goals which, as noted above, is vital to its legitimating function. This particular policy concept includes changes to local government powers and town planning regulations (to involve local neighbourhoods), and 'opening up public services' (Cabinet Office 2011a) to enable private companies and the voluntary sector to provide more services on behalf of the state, alongside a range of initiatives to encourage active citizenship. These diffuse notions not only combine into a nebulous overall framework, but moreover their understanding of society is fluid and often focused at such a local level that it may be seen to encourage people to care for other 'people like us' but to undermine a more expansive notion of societal-level care which was epitomised in the Beveridge image of the welfare state and the NHS.

---

have resulted in a wave of governance features throughout the NHS. At the centre of these are the changes to the management of risk, knowledge and performance brought under the 'umbrella' of clinical governance (Flynn 2002). Following Moran, the governance agenda in the NHS can be read as a policitisation of and reaction against institutional failures such as the Bristol Royal Infirmary dysfunction (see chapter 5), and the weaving together of pre-existing trends to counteract spiralling litigation, a 'postcode lottery' in accessibility and standards of care, and increasing pressure on scarce resources (Brown 2008b). The compelling force of the governance agenda can be partly understood through its ideological presentation as an answer to these multiple and serious problems. Though, as discussed elsewhere in this book, whether such governance constitutes an enabling framework or is merely a guise of increasing, rather than devolved, command-and-control is highly contestable (Sheaff and Pilgrim 2006).

Risk – the ideology of ideologies

The predominance of governance within recent health policy is furthermore bound up in its prospective ability to manage risk. As stated above, *all* ideology, at its core, combines considerations of what is normatively good, correct and desirable, and a methodology of how this end is most effectively pursued in a more practical sense (Eatwell 1993: 13). As a heightened awareness of risk and uncertainty has become a defining phenomenon of late-modern society (Beck 1992; Furedi 2002) and health care (Alaszewski and Brown 2007), so has the potency of ideologies which offer means of countering or managing risk been enhanced. In turn, by recognising and seeking to counter risks, policy makers increase public awareness of these phenomena and add credence to their 'reality' and problematic nature (Bröer 2007).

It is this understanding of ideology and its practical implications which helps make apparent the fallacy of assertions that an end point of ideology has been reached (Bell 1960), or that real ideological struggle is a thing of the past (Fukuyama 1992). Although in some senses it would seem that Fukuyama (1992) is correct to note that the global capitalist hegemony has emerged with *relatively* low amounts of current contestation in the West (radical Islamism and sustainable environmentalism being two notable problems for this thesis), ideologies at the paradigmatic or grand narrative level have continued to be created. As we note in box 8.4, some argue that it is the very demise of the 'left–right' political spectrum within nation-states, not least the UK, that provided the platform for *risk* to develop as a decisive narrative around which recent political and policy events can be understood and future responses organised (Furedi 2005; Alaszewski and Brown 2007).

Box 8.4   The demise of left and right: the need for a 'new morality'

For much of the post-war period until the 1980s, party politics was fought along a left–right spectrum, rooted in perceptions of class interests and contrasted in terms of economic intervention – with the social democracy and One Nation Conservatism towards the left committed to state interventionism and welfare politics. In the 1980s this left–right positioning became more starkly polarised, with Thatcherite neo-liberalism (committed to reducing the size of the state) contrasted against the continued social democracy of the Labour Party.

More recently, party politics has converged around the centre – with little or no debate about class interests and a general consensus about government intervention in the economy.

As a result, parties need new ideologies around which they can mobilise support and differentiate themselves from their opponents. The 'Compassionate Conservatism' of Iain Duncan-Smith was one example of post-left–right morality (though with heavy echoes of One Nation Toryism). Arguably though, *risk* has emerged as one of the most potent tools for defining moral ground within the vacuum created by the end of explicit left–right discussions in politics.

Risk is arguably the most high-profile example of a symbolic, emotive policy concept which has increasingly been used as an ideological tool of legitimation – mobilising consensus around reconstructions of norms and values. The politics of fear (Furedi 2005) are thus a potent means of legitimating action which would otherwise be seen as running contrary to popular norms and vales – anti-terrorist legislation, referred to above, being one clear example. Risk has been peculiarly effective because its apparently scientific, actuarial basis would seem to place it beyond politics and moral questioning (Horlick-Jones 2005) – even though notions of risk and blame are deeply moral considerations (Douglas 1992). One apparent case in point is the changes to the nature of clinical practice and autonomy via the introduction of clinical governance and modifications to the role of the General Medical Council (see boxes 6.1 and 7.2). An agenda of countering medical risk to the public – as politicised through Bristol, Shipman, Alder Hey (Alaszewski 2002) and their 'emblematic' effect on the public imagination (Butler and Drakeford

2005) – has enabled a diminution of clinician power which would normally have been resisted with the utmost vigour by the British Medical Association and other professional bodies. Yet the ideological tool of risk has mobilised, or forced, a 'consensus' to emerge as to the appropriateness of limiting clinical freedom.

Risk is being applied in this context as an apparently politically neutral concept, its acceptance achieved by the politicisation of fear (Furedi 2005: 132), yet its effect, paradoxically, is the depoliticisation of everything else (Pieterman 2005). The 'heuristics of fear' (Jonas 1984) have emerged to fill the ideological vacuum left after the demise of left–right political discourse (Giddens 1994) and political attention has therefore shifted towards safety and risk. Risk-aversion, as an apparent universalised moral basis for policy (Furedi 2005: 137), obstructs political debate in that proposals based on this premise are seemingly indisputable. In this way, issues surrounding health care become distanced from discussions of interests and power due to the ostensibly 'neutral' language of risk (Jayasuriya 2001).

Choice – the provision of real alternatives or mere 'spin'

Alongside risk, choice has become a defining concept by which health policy in the English NHS is increasingly framed (Department of Health 2005b) – especially following the Darzi Review (Darzi 2008b). The development of a consumer-oriented worldview, alongside a continuing esteem of the invisible hand of the market and its ability to drive quality through competition (Le Grand 2007), are integral ideological asumptions behind this recent agenda. Competition (via the 'internal market') and an overt focus on price and efficiency were seen by policy makers as distinctly unpopular amongst the public (Department of Health 1997). Choice, on the other hand, could be said to represent the palatable face of competition – likely to be more popular as a rhetorical tool amongst the public, regardless of the similarities in practice. Whereas 'choice' in health care 'becomes a "new paternalism" in which the availability of a patient-centred service, a high priority for users, does not figure on the agenda of providers' (Taylor-Gooby 2008: 165), its *conceptual* capacity to focus attention on service-users and their needs, rhetorically fulfilling government objectives of a patient-centred NHS, is believed by policy makers to be ideologically compelling.

It would be overly simplistic to suggest that the choice agenda, as it has recently been articulated by policy makers, is completely analogous with the internal market of the 1990s. Yet the underlying similarities nevertheless illuminate one fundamental role of ideology discussed earlier in the chapter – the linking of practical policy functions with norms and values. That the proposals in practice – of competition and choice – are so similar, and yet the rhetoric is quite different, illustrates the potential utility of ideology in winning legitimacy for policy enactments in a manner which is quite distanced from substantive considerations. This potential for gaps to exist between the ideological process of framing or 'spin' (oriented towards a goal of legitimation) and the practical substance of the policy (oriented towards technical effectiveness) underlines the way in which ideology may well generate ambivalence, distraction and correspondingly irrational policy (at the substantive level).

The 'choice' agenda, associated economically with competition and the market, is politically attributable to Third-Way notions of decentralisation and localised democracy (see chapter 7). Both these ideological bases may be legitimate and useful in framing and bounding policy making, yet localised choice and service responsiveness towards this may be highly incompatible with the problems of geographical variations (postcode lotteries) referred to above. In this sense ideological pragmatism, the natural conclusion of a reactive and evolving ideology (as discussed above), may only make for increasingly inconsistent and counter-productive policy. Once again, this can be seen as a result of defensive and adversarial party politics – one in which a highly critical rather than consensus-based democratic system greatly inhibits the possibility for substantively rational decision making.

The inconsistencies of this pragmatic and responsive ideology, as with the spin which surrounds it, have become increasingly apparent to the public. Here the negative connotations attached to ideology (epitomised by the 'spin doctor') act to undermine the legitimacy of governments. Spin is a vague concept, loosely applied in the media and general parlance. However, it is possible to be more specific about its usage by considering it as strategic, perlocutionary influence directed towards norms. In a Habermasian sense (Habermas 1984), strategic action is aimed not so much at enhancing shared understanding through considered debate but more cynically at achieving specific goals – not least legitimacy. Perlocutionary communication is one method of doing this, using language and broader communication to engineer certain psychological reactions across the public sphere. This approach is thus able to influence public opinion and attach practical policies to certain normative notions in order

---

Box 8.5   Ideology functioning on many levels – 'micro'- ideology around intermediate care

Gramsci distinguished between 'science', mass ideology and more practical/common-sense praxis. From this we can suggest that ideology exists and functions on a number of different levels:

- Ideology as prevailing hegemony (for example, capitalist liberal-democracy)
- Ideology as party-political (for example, New Labour versus Conservative)
- Ideology as practical and policy-orientated (for example, intermediate-care – see below).

Intermediate care

Problem   Insufficient care in community / primary care sector and therefore high use of acute beds by older people. This resulted in long-term bed-blocking and a 'revolving door syndrome' – whereby older people were discharged only to deteriorate and be readmitted.

Ideologies invoked   Keeping older people independent and in their own homes (in the community) is the preferred means of organising care; partnership between health and social services.

Policy created   Funding and providing 'Intermediate care' services, offering incentives for partnership working between health and social services to enable many more older people to be cared for in their own homes – Community Care (Delayed Discharge etc) Act 2003.

---

to gain support – despite the gap between rhetoric and substance. This conception of spin is most (in)famously associated with Alistair Campbell, the communications and strategy aide to Tony Blair from 1997 to 2003.

Comment

While the concept of ideology is difficult to define, it clearly plays a major role in the development of policies. It provides the legitimacy for policies and it frames, and in the process simplifies, complex conditions so that policy makers can focus on the key 'issues' and decisions. However, in facilitating and legitimating action it effectively compromises the rationality of policy making.

KEY POINTS

- The concept of ideology is nebulous and slippery to define. In practice though, and in relation to health policy, ideologies can most usefully be thought of as notions which link norms and values to practical action.
- Ideology performs a number of vital roles for policy makers: enabling legitimacy by associating practical action with normative 'rightness'; bounding rationality and thus prioritising certain concerns over others, therefore enabling action amidst a multitude of complex possibilities; and by framing problems through a particular ideological lens, policy makers are directed towards specific interests and actors.
- Ideology functions on multiple levels, in one sense being invented and used by policy makers as a means of gaining support. Yet ideology also transcends policy decisions, forming a more fundamental paradigm upon which decisions are considered and in which evaluations of rationality, appropriateness and effectiveness are made.
- Rational policy making is compromised by ideology: informed, reasoned debate and decision making are hindered by the warping influence of spin and a pandering towards populism – more fundamental ideologies/paradigms limit what is deemed possible, therefore making policy makers docile to certain assumptions, precluding a broader consideration of interests and potentially effective options.
- The palpable 'dark side' of ideology, where rhetoric becomes divorced from substance, is apparent in the way bureaucracies handle risk – there is a tendency to prioritise the minimising of risk to the institution ahead of concerns of risk to the public (Rothstein 2006). This pathology is also palpable around the notion of 'spin' – a tool used by policy makers towards legitimation but which paradoxically has recently been perceived as undermining the legitimacy of political institutions and parties.
- While in the long term governments are able to create new assumptions about the role of the NHS and effective policy towards health, in the short term new ideas are always influenced by what has gone before – on the one hand reacting against what

has been seen as problematic, on the other hand curtailed by what is seen as possible and do-able.

- Following a demise of left–right welfare politics, new ideological concepts have arisen which in many ways are highly sophisticated. Risk in particular has been seen as useful in resonating with the public and thus legitimating policy. This concept also provides an effective way of bounding policy logic and pointing decision-makers to certain solutions.

9

The impact of the media on health policy making

AIMS

To examine the ways in which the mass media influence and shape the making of health policy

OBJECTIVES

- To consider the nature of modern mass media and its role as a source of knowledge about the world and policy issues
- To examine the ways in which the mass media influence the types of issues, knowledge and relationships in the policy process
- To explore the ways in which media reporting creates pressure for immediate action, limiting the scope for rational policy making.

We argued in the first part of this book that rationality is both an important objective and major justification of policy making in contemporary democratic societies. However, to be rational, policy making needs to be grounded in knowledge, whether this is knowledge of the most effective means of achieving a specified end (instrumental rationality), of the interests and views of groups involved and affected by specific policies (communicative rationality), or of the nature and causes of policy failure (retrospective rationality). While policy makers can access knowledge through using experts or collecting their own evidence, they operate in a social context in which the mass media have become a major, if not the major, source of knowledge about social issues and how they should be addressed. As we will show in this chapter the mass media have come to play a decisive role in the formation of health policy.

9.1 The mass media, knowledge and mediated representation

Social changes: the decline of face-to-face relationships as the source of knowledge

The most reliable and concrete source of knowledge is direct personal experience. In pre-modern, small-scale societies in which intimate face-to-face interactions were prominent, direct experience provided a reliable source for much of the knowledge needed for everyday decision making and life (Beattie 1966). Since the technological and social changes that started in the fifteenth century, such small-scale societies have largely been replaced by large-scale interconnected urban-based societies. In this context, knowledge based on direct personal experience is inevitably limited and needs to be supplemented by indirect sources. Indirect sources were available in pre-modern societies but these tended to be personal – via third parties who witnessed events – or religious – such as religious experts, oracles or texts that offered understanding of phenomena that could be directly experienced (see, for example, Evans-Pritchard 1976). The increasing complexity of modern societies means that direct experience is more limited and traditional sources of information via third parties or religious texts are not accepted as authoritative or trustworthy. In most contemporary societies, printed and electronic media provide the main source of knowledge about the world that exists beyond the scope of personal experience. 'Because only a small handful of events can ever be experienced by individuals at first hand, we inevitably rely on the mass media to inform us about events beyond our immediate grasp' (Negrine 1994: 3).

The mass media provide the basic '"informational building blocks" . . . [which] determine the limits of our knowledge and our perception of events and their causes' (Negrine 1994: 3). To be convincing, such building blocks must be seen as trustworthy. The mass media tend to combine two processes in developing this sense of trustworthiness:

- *Truthfulness* The development of formal scientific methods influenced the emergence of the mass media and shaped approaches to scrutinising and assessing the truthfulness of sources of evidence. Thus newspapers employ professional journalists who scrutinise and evaluate sources of information, and editors who select and publish those stories which they see as having public and audience interest (see, for example, Kitzinger 1999). The rigour of such scrutiny varies from the full scientific rigour of peer-reviewed journals to the relative openness and accessibility of the internet.

However, as Riesch and Spiegelhalter (2011) noted, even when the source of information is as authoritative as a press release from a scientific research group, journalists and editors critically evaluate the evidence and make their own interpretation. Thus, such processes tend to be impersonal, critical and technical and, as Mairal (2011) noted, newspaper articles often include precise and technical data to establish the general or abstract truth underpinning specific reports.

- *Authenticity* While the existence of systematic scrutiny enhances the potential truthfulness of material in the media, it does not overcome, and indeed creates, a distance between the events being reported and individuals accessing the reports. Such reports are indirect representations of past events. To overcome such distancing, indirect representations need to be personalised and one way of doing this is through the 'eye witness'. Mairal (2011) has argued that the earliest development of journalism, such as the reporting of the Lisbon earthquake of 1755, combined technical and abstract accounts of events with highly personal eye-witness descriptions. This narrative matrix was evident not only in factual accounts but also in fictional or imaginative recreations of events such as Daniel Defoe's depiction of the London Plague, which we discuss in box 9.1. The development of new technology such as photography and television has created new ways of overcoming the depersonalising effects of distance. Pollard (2011) noted in her analysis of the impact of media coverage of the 9/11 attack on the World Trade Center in New York that television coverage of the disaster meant that images and the associated trauma were directly accessed by viewers, who collectively became eye witnesses to the events. The emotional, concrete and personal experience involved in witnessing events through the media provides authenticity to such indirect representations of events.

Journalistic representations of reality are the major source of knowledge about the world in secular democratic societies such as the UK. These representations tend to be treated as truthful and trustworthy. Schutz (1964: 33–53), in his analysis of everyday social experience and knowledge, argued that when individuals do not have direct personal experience based on face-to-face contact they have to rely on generalised abstractions – typifications or stereotypes – to make sense of people and events (p. 42). Thus, they are likely to treat their own direct experiences as more credible and trustworthy. However, such is the effectiveness of the mass media that in some

---

Box 9.1   Daniel Defoe and the London Plague

Context   Daniel Defoe was born in London in 1659 or 1660. As a young child he lived through the 1665 plague. In 1704 he published an eye-witness account of the 1703 storm that devastated London. Following the reappearance of plague in Marseille in 1720, he wrote *A Journal of the Plague Year*, an account of the London Plague of 1665 (Defoe 1722).

Purpose of the account   To make Londoners aware of the risk of a new plague, and to help them minimise the impact of such a plague by drawing on the experiences and lessons of the 1665 Plague.

Eye-witness account   The book purported to be a contemporary diary and the record of the experiences of a merchant who was '*a citizen who continued all the while in London*' during the Plague year of 1665.

Technical evidence   The book combined a highly personal and emotional account of the plague with technical details about the ways in which the disease spread and the response to this spread.

Narrative matrix   While the account was fictional, the combination of the personal feelings and technical detail created a sense of reality and an ethnography providing the reader with a feeling of what it must have been like to live through the 1665 London Plague.

---

circumstances individuals treat representation in the mass media as more trustworthy than their own direct experiences, even where such representations are fictional. For example, Hughes, Kitzinger and Murdock (2004: 258–9) have examined the way in which Mary Shelley's gothic novel *Frankenstein* has become a generally accepted representation of science exceeding its limits and producing creations that it cannot control. Kitzinger (2004) also examined the ways in which the media emphasised stranger danger, i.e. the threat of sexual abuse to young children, showing how it reinforced audience stereotypes and masked the more common threat of abuse from those known to the child. Furthermore, as we show in box 9.2, Philo (1999) argued that media representations of people with mental health are treated as truer than personal experiences.

Box 9.2   Mediated representations of mental illness

Context   In the early 1990s, the Glasgow Media Group (Philo 1999) examined the ways in which press and television media represented people with mental illness and set up a series of focus groups to examine the ways in which audiences interpreted such media representations.

Media representation   During a period of one month, the researchers identified 562 representations of mental illness which fell into five categories: violence to others; harm to self; advice; criticism of ways in which mental illness was defined; and 'comic' images. The most common representation was that of people with mental illness as violent and this dominated the front pages; more sympathetic representations tended to be in specialist sections such as the health pages.

Audience reception   In their audience research, the Group generally found 'that personal experience is a much stronger influence on belief than messages which are given by the media' (Philo 1999: 56). In the case of mental illness, the reverse was the case. The audience tended to accept representations of people with mental illness as violent, often citing fictional characters such as Trevor Jordache in the soap opera *Brookside*, who was referred to in the popular press as 'psycho Trevor'. Participants in the focus group used him as an example of 'what a mentally ill person was really like'. Furthermore, 21 per cent of the participants in the study were people who had personal experiences of people with mental illness and had not experienced any violence. Yet even this group accepted the media representation of people with mental illness as violent. One woman who had visited a patient for twenty-five years and stated 'Oh aye – everyday I was up visiting, I never saw any violence and he was in a big open ward' yet associated mental illness with violence, citing horror films such as *Nightmare on Elm Street* as the source of her belief (Philo 1999: 56).

Changing nature of policy making and the impact of the mass media

The nature and context of policy making has changed over time, as we argued in chapter 1, and the main aspects of such changes are the increasing distance between key participants in the process and the impersonality of key parts of the process.

In England the initial development of a more democratic system in the eighteenth century did not substantially disrupt the intimate and personalised relationships between key participants in the policy-making process as government remained small-scale and informal, and the franchise was highly restricted. During this golden period of parliamentary democracy, MPs often had direct and personal relations with relatively small electorates and played an important role in policy making – for example, reforming mental health legislation in the early nineteenth century was initiated by MPs' investigations into conditions in Bedlam and private madhouses (Jones 1993).

This golden age of Parliament coincided with the development of journalism and the mass media. While participants within the policy process did not require indirect representations as they had face-to-face relations, most of the population was excluded from the political and policy-making process and for these people the media provided representations of political decision making. Governments sought to control representations through censorship and other forms of control (Wheeler 1997: 3), but the media proved adept at evading such control. For example, satirical cartoons – first developed in sixteenth-century Germany as a way of providing critical representations of religious opponents – in eighteenth-century Britain provided representations of a corrupt political elite. In a cartoon published in 1787 James Gillray satirised the British political establishment, using monstrous claws to represent the greed of George III and Queen Charlotte (Wright and Evans 1851: vii). As box 9.3 shows, the role of the media in promoting alternative representations of social and political relations can also be seen in the role of the *Lancet* in promoting medical reform.

While it is self-evident that the mass media play an important role in contemporary politics and policy making, the precise nature of this role is less clear. If the mass media were a neutral source of knowledge, then it would be one source amongst many, but, as Wheeler noted, the 'mass media have become key political actors' (1997: 239) and exert their own independent influence on politics and policy making. As the central source and location for exchange of representations, media can play an active role in creating the knowledge used within policy making.

Box 9.3 *The Lancet* and medical reform

Context At the end of the eighteenth century the medical profession was divided into three separate groups: apothecaries (tradesmen), surgeons (craftsmen) and physicians (gentlemen). The emergence of the middle classes, especially in the industrial and urban North of England, created the demand for a general medical practitioner. The 1815 Apothecaries Act created an inferior and subordinate position for General Practitioners and, for over forty years, together with surgeons, they campaigned for equal status with physicians through the formation of a single unified state-regulated profession, which they partially achieved in the 1858 Medical Registration Act (Parry and Parry 1976: 104–30).

The medical reform movement The General Practitioners and surgeons had to challenge the existing representation of the hierarchy as a natural reflection of different skills and expertise. In this they were allied to the wider contemporary radical reform movement that drew on media representation of corrupt church and legal institutions and corrupt electoral systems, resulting in the extension of the franchise through the 1832 Reform Bill. The medical reform movement developed its own campaigning bodies, the Provincial Medical and Surgical Association (later to become the British Medical Association), and its own journal, the *Lancet*.

Undermining the medical establishment The *Lancet* was first published on 5 October 1823. Its founder, Thomas Wakley, a surgeon, intended his journal to have a distinctive matrix: scientific instruction plus medical reform. He noted that 'A lancet can be an arched window to let in the light or it can be a sharp surgical instrument to cut out the dross and I intend to use it in both senses' (The Lancet.com n.d.: 1). Wakley used the *Lancet* to represent the established medical corporations, such as the Royal College of Physicians, as corrupt, self-serving and requiring modernisation. For example, in 1841 he stated that 'The Council of the College of Surgeons remains an irresponsible, unreformed monstrosity in the midst of English institutions – an antediluvian relic of all . . . that is most despotic and revolting, iniquitous and insulting, on the face of the Earth' (Wakley 1841: 246).

9.2 Structuring knowledge through the mass media: alternative views

Analysts of the mass media as an independent and distinctive contributor to policy and policy making fall into two main groups: those who see the media acting for or on behalf of particular social interests and groups; and those who focus on the distinctive and autonomous dynamics of the mass media.

The media and dominant interests

Marxist commentators have focused on the role of the mass media in protecting dominant interests in society. This approach can be traced back to Marx himself, who argued that institutions such as the mass media reflected the interests of capitalists and acted to promote the institutions of capitalism, such as private property. He noted that: 'The class which has the means of production at its disposal has control at the same time over the production and distribution of ideas of their age' (Marx and Engels 1977: 64). Thus Marxists have argued that there is a systematic bias in the media with the suppression of interests which would threaten the status quo.

Supporting evidence for this type of analysis can be found in the newspaper presentation of political events. For example, the 1980s was a period of heightened political conflict in the UK during which a radical Conservative Government led by Margaret Thatcher sought to make fundamental reforms to the public sector, including the NHS, and to reduce the power of trade unions. This Government established close working relationships with the media, for example enabling News International and its chairman Rupert Murdoch to add the broadsheets *The Times* and *The Sunday Times* to its existing portfolio, which included the tabloids the *Sun* and the *News of the World*. These papers supported the Government and its reform programme. In the 1979 election, the *Sun* urged its readers to vote for Mrs Thatcher as the 'only radical proposals being put to you are being put by Maggie Thatcher and her Tory team' (Wheeler 1997: 67); in 1992 when the Conservative Party won the closely fought election, the *Sun* claimed credit for the victory with the headline 'IT'S THE SUN WOT WON IT' (Kingdom 1999: 206); and in 1997, Tony Blair, the leader of the Labour Party, established a close relationship with Rupert Murdoch, resulting in a shift in the allegiances of the *Sun*, when on 18 March 1997, the headline proclaimed that 'THE SUN BACKS BLAIR' (Kingdom 1999: 207).

Media bias is most evident in events that have a clear political relevance, where public attention can be deflected from the problems of the political elite towards threatening but marginal groups in society. Cohen (2002) in his classic study of folk devils and moral panics explored the media coverage of Mods and Rockers which began with coverage of the disturbances in Clacton in Easter 1964 (2002: 32). The development of hostile stereotypes of Mods and Rockers and the use of seaside disturbances as evidence of major moral failing in society took place within the context of a Conservative Government which had been tainted by scandal, such as the Profumo affair, and hung onto power until it was compelled to call a general election in October 1964. For Cohen, there was a systematic bias which favoured established and powerful groups – for example, he noted that newspapers such as the *Daily Mail* and *Daily Telegraph* counteracted the representation of the police as racist following the Macpherson Report which had identified 'institutionalized racism' in the Metropolitan police (Cohen 2002: xi). In contrast, powerless, marginalised groups could be stereotyped as morally threatening, with these depictions used to justify repressive policies. Cohen argued that in the early 1990s Conservative politicians struggling for popularity 'cynically constructed the single mother as a potent moral threat', encouraging media representation of 'single mothers as irresponsible adults and ineffective parents . . . to legitimize and entrench shrinking public provision' (Cohen 2002: xviii). The development of media constructions such as folk devils and the resulting moral panics implies that these issues are socially significant and within the scope of 'high politics' (Walt 1994) – so important that they require an immediate government response.

Given the high profile of media owners, such as Rupert Murdoch, and well-published events such as the *Sun*'s support for the Conservative Party in 1992, there is a strong perception that parts of the mass media are biased towards the interests of their owners and to political parties and policies that favour these interests. However, it is difficult to systematically identify and measure media bias without, as Cohen (2002) did in the case of Mods and Rockers, undertaking a detailed independent analysis of the individuals and events as a base line against which to identify such bias.

Sanders, Marsh and Ward (1993) suggest an alternative way of exploring media bias. They compared the ways in which different newspapers reported on the same news – official government economic statistics such as levels of unemployment, economic growth or balance of payments on international trade. They found that, between elections, newspaper content did to some extent reflect overall editorial policy, with those papers with stated support for the Conservative Government tending to report news more positively than those with different leanings. However, the differences were relatively small, and on some issues, such as reporting news of balance of payments, pro-Government papers were actually more negative than other papers – with all papers reporting negatively on unemployment and balance of payments issues. The reporting in the two main Murdock papers that purported to support the Conservative Government was either negative (*The Times*) or relatively neutral (*Sun*). However, in the run-up to a general election, there was a marked change. The editorial policy strongly affected the coverage and presentation of economic news. Thus the difference between pro-Conservative and pro-Labour papers was marked, with papers such as the *Daily Telegraph*, the *Daily Mail* and the *Sun* emphasising the positive aspects of economic information and the *Mirror* emphasising the negative. Thus, when important high-profile issues were at stake, as at general elections or during periods of internal and external conflict, British national newspapers did overtly take sides and structured the ways they presented information.

While simple measures of bias may not support a direct and overt relationship between media representations and dominant interests within contemporary societies, Marxist commentators argue that the relationship is deeper, more complex and essentially hidden. Broader cultural representations legitimate the current status quo by persuading deprived and excluded groups that it is a fair and just society. This acts to undermine challenges to the status quo. For example Couldry (2000: 127) argued that negative stereotypes of protesters imply that ordinary citizens cannot alter their circumstances through their own actions. Thus, as Hall (1991) described, the representations of current social reality are ideological and therefore operate at subconscious as well as conscious levels.

Habermas (1989) has argued that the media relationship with the state has changed over time. As the power of capitalists and the state grew in the nineteenth century, so the scope for the media to provide space for interactions and exchanges between private citizens was reduced and the media increasingly acted as a forum for organised interests, as we noted in chapter 7. However, if agents such as the media are to operate effectively to protect the interests of dominant groups, then they must act to conceal these relationships. Thus, Althusser argued that marginalised and deprived groups are only truly disempowered when they are persuaded that they are free to make choices and enjoy the opportunities afforded to the privileged: 'They must be induced to "live" their exploitation and oppression in such a way that they do not experience or represent to themselves their position as one in which they are exploited and oppressed' (Althusser cited in Wheeler 1997: 25). This concealment means that the media must appear to allow for the articulation of competing interests and views. However, in reality the media always favour dominant groups and interests in society.

Reforms such as development of state health care in Britain present an interesting challenge to Marxist analysts as these represent altruistic welfare reforms which redistributed wealth to benefit deprived and marginalised groups. However, Vicente Navarro (1978) used a Marxist perspective to challenge traditional accounts of health reforms in Britain, arguing that they were minimalist concessions that actually reinforced class differentials such as inequalities in health.

The internal dynamic of the media

While the mass media provide links between individuals and institutions, they are, or appear to be, independent from those individuals and institutions, operating on the basis of their own internal logic and dynamic. To attract and sustain an audience in an increasingly competitive environment a media outlet such as a newspaper needs to identify those stories its readers want to read, select and simplify complex reality so it is comprehensible to potential readers, and present stories in such a way that readers find them interesting and relevant.

The process of identifying items to be included in media outlets to which there is restricted access involves selecting issues which are considered important. In the case of newspapers, such filtering is generally done by journalists who may use their tacit knowledge to identify potentially interesting or newsworthy items. As Kitzinger (2006: 253) has argued, because media outlets such as newspapers are complex organisations operating in competitive environments with limited budgets and tight (often daily) deadlines, such selections have to be made quickly, with little time for reflection. However, journalists do reflect on the criteria they use and try to make these explicit. Hetherington (cited in Negrine 1994: 121–2), a former editor of the *Guardian*, a quality UK newspaper, indicated that he selected events on the basis of their social, political, economic and human 'significance' and their potential interest to readers in terms of drama or excitement, surprise and unexpectedness, the personalities or celebrities affected/involved, potential salaciousness such as sex scandal or crime, and numbers involved or hurt. Negrine (1994: 122) suggests that such criteria mean newsworthiness tends to be defined in terms of events that threaten or disrupt the peace and stability of liberal democracy – particularly, as we discussed in chapter 5 – disasters.

The newsworthiness of an issue or story reflects both the dynamic of the media – i.e. the need to have a story that makes an impact – and the values of both journalists and their audiences (Kitzinger 2006: 255–8). Thus, events which take time to unfold and have an impact are not likely to be considered newsworthy. Protest groups against Genetically Modified (GM) crops in Britain only got media coverage when they dressed in white boiler suits and ripped out crops, creating powerful photographic images that linked the potential harm of GM crops to the actual harm of the Chernobyl disaster (Kitzinger 2006: 256). Similarly, vCJD, the human form of mad cow disease, only became newsworthy when journalists could interview people with the disease (Kitzinger 2006: 256). Events that cause high levels of harm within a short period of time, such as a train crash or a tsunami, are newsworthy, but only if the victims can be directly linked in some way to the audience (Kitzinger 2006: 256–7). Thus the terrorist bombs which exploded in London in July 2005, killing 52 people, and the death of 179 British soldiers in Iraq received major news coverage in the British media; in contrast, Iraqi casualties, which the Iraqi Health Minister in 2006 estimated at over 100 a day, received minimal British media coverage. The precise identity of the person involved affects the newsworthiness as well as the moral dimension of the event (Kitzinger 2006: 256–8), thus newsworthiness is increased if an event affects a celebrity and their actions are somehow reprehensible, or if a person or institution can be blamed for failing to protect an innocent victim – for example, not protecting a child from serious harm as in the Baby P case (Glendinning and Tran 2008).

Newsworthiness also relates to the ways in which a story can be framed. As Galtung and Ruge (cited in Negrine 1989: 120) argued, newsworthy events are likely to relate to issues that readers find familiar but that are somehow distinctive or unexpected. The framing of a story establishes its familiarity often by linking it to a 'similar' well-known iconic event which is the defining example or anchor for subsequent events. Thus, the Watergate scandal, in which the arrest of five men for breaking into the Democratic National Committee headquarters in the Watergate complex led to the resignation of President Richard Nixon in 1974, has become the iconic event for political scandal and cover-up. As we discussed in chapter 5, in the field of mental health the killing on Finsbury Park Station on December 1992 of Jonathan Zito, a newly wed musician, by Christopher Clunis, who had been discharged from mental hospital (Ritchie Inquiry 1994), has become the iconic event signifying the dangerousness of people with mental illness. Warner (2006: 225) indicated that Christopher Clunis has become the iconic 'high-risk' figure in the media and, through this representation, an archetype for the social workers.

While certain icons tend to be dominant, there is scope for alternative representation or different ways of framing the same events. As Eldridge noted 'the media occupy space which is constantly being contested' (1993: 20). In our discussion of interest groups in chapter 6, we noted the ways in which pressure groups tried to use the media to persuade audiences, especially key policy makers, of their definition of the nature of problems and solutions, and therefore to frame events in these terms. In box 6.5 we explored the limited success of groups such as Mind and the Royal College of Psychiatrists in challenging the dominant representation of people with mental illness in terms of the 'Clunis' frame. In some circumstances the challenge to the dominant frame comes from key policy makers. As we show in box 9.4, in the mid-1980s policy makers wanted to challenge the dominant initial representation of HIV/AIDS as a disease of marginalised groups, i.e. gay men and intravenous drug users, and therefore not a threat to the wider heterosexual population.

The existence of iconic stories and their repeated use to frame events create templates that journalists apply when interpreting and presenting new events. Kitzinger (2004: 72–3) argued that the defining elements of such templates are:

- key events that are recalled and reused;
- their use as an explanation of current events and as evidence of an underlying persistent problem;
- single primary meaning that excludes alternative explanation and debate.

Kitzinger (2004: 73) suggested that such templates are powerful and difficult to challenge. In the process of becoming a template, the complexity of a situation is simplified and distorted – the event is reduced to its essence but the precise meaning may subtly change as the key event is linked to, and interpreted within, the light of new events. Kitzinger (2004) explored the ways in which the 1987

Box 9.4   Framing HIV/AIDS: A gay disease or a threat to heterosexuals? (Beharrell 1993; Miller and Williams 1993)

Context   Towards the end of the 1970s, a new lethal disease started to affect gay men, particularly on the west coast of the USA, before spreading to Europe. In England, Terrence Higgins, who died in July 1982, was one of the first victims. His partner and friends established the Terrence Higgins Trust to promote awareness of the disease and prevent its spread.

Media coverage: the gay disease   In the early stages of the epidemic up to 1985, the Government played a relatively passive role, collecting scientific evidence on the nature of the new disease. From the start, the AIDS epidemic was newsworthy and became increasingly so when the victims included celebrities such as the pop star Freddie Mercury, who died in November 1991, and the ballet dancer Rudolf Nureyev, who died in January 1993. While the media did recognise 'innocent victims', e.g. haemophiliacs who had been infected by contaminated blood products, the main emphasis was on individuals, especially gay men, who through their (immoral) lifestyle had contributed to their own misfortune.

Contesting the dominant representation   In 1986 the Government acknowledged that HIV was a major public health problem and initiated a health promotion campaign to challenge public perceptions of the disease. This campaign was based on the representation of HIV as a sexually transmitted disease that could be prevented through behaviour changes such as 'safe sex'. In the late 1980s the Government had some success in reframing media presentations that reflected ownership, journalistic and marketing strategies. The owner of the Mirror Group, Robert Maxwell, was a co-founder of the National AIDS Trust, and the *Mirror* campaigned for compensation for infected haemophiliacs. On World AIDS day in 1988 the paper endorsed the health promotion message that the only way to stop the spread of HIV was 'through information, education and changes in human behaviour'. In contrast, a *Sun* column emphasised that the disease 'belonged' to gays 'since homosexuals whether they like it or not (and they don't) – DID start it'. The audience also played a role in shaping editorial policy. For example the *Daily Express* and *Daily Mail* were both tabloids oriented towards a conservative middle-class audience and both had a strong editorial policy that rejected the heterosexual framing of HIV/AIDS and attacked the health promotion campaign. An editorial in the *Daily Express* on 14 February 1990 stated that 'The government's persistence with [health promotion aimed at heterosexuals] can now be explained only by ministerial sensitivity towards not just the homosexual lobby but also wantonly alarmist doctors.' However, the framing was not consistent – for example, medical correspondents in both papers drew attention to the rapid increase in the number of cases resulting from heterosexual transmission (*Daily Mail*, 12 April 1990). The involvement of celebrities also had an impact on framing. For example, Princess Diana's involvement with AIDS sufferers was negatively received by some tabloid papers, and the *Mail on Sunday* (1 September 1991) carried a story which asked 'Could she really want to go down in history as the patron saint of sodomy?'. In contrast, the *Sun*, which started with chauvinist coverage of her involvement in 1989 was, by 1991, referring to her 'Vigil at hospital' in terms of 'Heartbroken Princess Diana wept last night after visiting a friend dying of AIDS in hospital' (23 August 1991).

Cleveland scandal became a media template for contested allegations of child sexual abuse, and the ways in which journalists and others used this template in the 1991 Orkney affair, as outlined in box 9.5.

As Kitzinger (2004) made clear, such templates often involve value judgements. Thus, in the case of the Cleveland template, the coverage of the story evoked empathy with the parents and presented negative images of incompetent and inhumane social workers. As in a morality play, the readers of the national newspapers were implicitly being invited to pass judgement and allocate blame and responsibility for the shocking events. However the moral of a story is not fixed – as we show in the case of the Lincolnshire sextuplets in box 9.6, it may change through claims and counterclaims.

The media play a key role in linking individuals and institutions in contemporary society – they structure the ways in which events and people are represented and the way knowledge about them is accessed. The relationship between the media and the rest of society is variable and depends on context. In some circumstances the owners of specific parts of the media or the government can and do exercise influence on the nature of mediated representations. However, the media have their own structure and dynamic. Through

Box 9.5   The Cleveland scandal: the development of a template for contested allegations of abuse

Context   The Maria Colwell case (1973) in which social services failed to prevent a seven-year-old girl from being killed by her stepfather was the 'child protection' template before being replaced by more recent disasters such as Victoria Climbié (2000) and Baby P (2007). However, in 1987 two local hospital paediatricians in Cleveland used an anal reflex dilation test to identify 121 children, from 51 families, who, they felt, showed evidence of sexual abuse. These children were taken into care by the local social service department.

Developing a new 'contested' abuse template   This case was different from that of Colwell. It involved multiple families and the evidence of harm was contested. The parents claimed there was a misdiagnosis and they were supported by the local Member of Parliament and police surgeons. The mass media accepted these claims with headlines such as 'Agony of families in sex abuse row' and all the children were returned to their parents (but since there was an embargo on media reporting of individual cases, there was no reporting of any continuing social services supervision).

Applying the template   In 1991, nine children from four families on the Orkney Islands were taken into social care for alleged abuse. The families again contested the proceedings. Most of the media used Cleveland as a template – for example, 'How the nightmare of Orkney ignored the lessons of Cleveland' (*Evening Standard* 4 April 1991). Only the *Guardian* accepted the claim of the Orkney social services that these were different cases, with the headline 'Orkney abuse case "unlike Cleveland"' (30 August 1991). The template involved a selective remembering of the Cleveland case, thus, while the key role of doctors and dispute between them was forgotten, the role of social workers was recalled and the template emphasised social work malpractice. Thus social workers were referred to in the media as 'child stealers' and 'neo-fascists' and the *Daily Mail* concluded that 'for the sake of all the broken-heart families, we must get rid of social workers and think again' (5 April 1991).

Box 9.6   Media and morality: the case of the Lincolnshire sextuplets

Context   On 19 May 1993, following IVF treatment in a local hospital, Mrs Vince, from Lincolnshire, gave birth to six live babies in Leeds.

Initial positive media coverage   On 20–21 May 1993, the birth was reported in the local evening paper and the story sold to a national tabloid, the *News of the World*. The coverage was positive and used a 'medical miracle' frame.

Negative coverage   On 22 May, the *Daily Mail* reframed the story with a front page headlined 'Bizarre life of six-baby parents'. The report included a comment from MP Robert Spink criticising the local health authority for authorising the IVF treatment. On 24 May most tabloids had reports on the sextuplets. The *Daily Express* had the headline 'Sextuplets to cost the taxpayers £800,000'. The coverage was critical, emphasising the irresponsibility of the parents, medical practitioners and Government in allowing this to happen

Government response to criticism   Tom Sackville, a junior minister of health, passed the blame. He emphasised that local doctors applied their clinical judgement and that health authorities 'should think carefully before providing fertility treatment to people without a stable family background'. He initiated a review of health authority practice.

---

the selection and framing of events and people, the media creates templates that are used to make moral judgements and to allocate blame and responsibility.

9.3 The relationship between the mass media and health policy makers: controlled or controlling

Trying to control the media template

As part of the implementation of health policy, the inner core of policy makers – ministers and their advisers – often seek to influence media representations. This is particularly evident in the case of public health where policy makers identify a form of behaviour that is harmful to the health of the population and seek to change public perceptions as part of the process of changing behaviours. As we noted above, the initial media representation of HIV/AIDS was that of a gay disease. In the mid-1980s health policy makers came to view the disease as one that was sexually transmitted and as a major threat to the whole population that could only be combated by a radical shift in sexual behaviour, i.e. safer sex. The Health Education Authority (HEA) led the Government campaign to change attitudes (see Beharrell 1993: 210–49). They launched a high-profile 'AIDS kills' campaign and used various tactics to change media representations. Such tactics included providing statistics that showed heterosexuals were also involved, though only the *Independent* (18 November 1989) carried the HEA statistics. Another tactic was to run television adverts based on personal testimonies of infected heterosexuals. Such personalised drama fitted well with the format of the tabloid press. For example one of the smaller UK tabloids, the *Daily Star,* included the following example: 'Alison is 24, rich and got AIDS from the man of her dreams . . . in a one-night stand several years ago – and now she's dying of AIDS . . . and now Alison lives with the ticking time-bomb of despair' (23 August 1990 cited in Beharrell 1993: 235). It is difficult to assess the effectiveness of such governmental attempts to change representations. In the case of HIV/AIDS, while the immediate impact of the HEA campaign may have been limited, in the longer term media representations did change with HIV/AIDS being represented as a sexually transmitted disease rather than as a specifically gay disease.

These media strategies relate to policy makers' efforts to shape the representation of issues and to foster beneficial coverage. However alongside these are more focused responses to events. As we noted in chapters 1 and 2, ministers are key policy makers who are the public face of policy making. Being a minister forms the apogee of a political career and politicians seek to build their reputation and enhance their career through policy making. However, politicians are not only responsible for policy which will shape the future, they are also responsible for the present and past, i.e. the effective delivery of policy. Thus failures in policy can damage their reputations, trustworthiness and authority. Such damage may not be limited to a specific area of government policy but may in serious cases undermine public confidence in the competence of the whole government. In the mid-1970s Barbara Castle's attempt to phase out pay beds in the NHS were undermined by media reports that in

1965 she had herself used private facilities in the NHS. The hostile media coverage weakened Castle's authority and public support and strengthened the negotiating position of the BMA so that Castle was forced to accept mediation from Lord Goodman, the Chairman of the Newspaper Proprietor's Association (Castle 1980). In the 1990s the Labour Government experienced similar problems. The Prime Minister Tony Blair had a private meeting with the Formula One boss Bernie Ecclestone. Within hours of the meeting Blair instructed the Minister responsible for public health to delay the implementation of the Europe-wide ban on tobacco advertising and sponsorship. Ecclestone also made a £1 million donation to the Labour Party (Oliver and Oakeshott 2008). Despite denials by the Prime Minister, the media presented the decision to exempt Formula One as a corrupt and sleazy transaction (*BBC News* 1997).

Given their vulnerability to critical media commentary, politicians are concerned to protect and enhance their reputations and are sensitive to media representations of their actions, especially when these are critical. Thus, ministers try to respond rapidly to any evidence of policy failures and shortcomings within their area of responsibility. As we noted in chapter 5, given the increasing role and complexity of government activities, such failures are inevitable and in the NHS there have been repeated disasters and scandals. The ministerial presentation of such failings tends to take a relatively predictable form – designed to establish the sincerity of the minister, to deflect blame and to take action. Thus ministerial statements include an acknowledgement of the unacceptability of the harm caused, a commitment to punish those individuals whose failing contributed to the disaster and an undertaking to identify the causes and rectify the systemic faults resulting in the disaster. In the case of Baby P, who was killed by his mother's partner and lodger even though he was the subject of a child protection plan, the Minister responsible, Ed Balls, stated:

> The whole nation has been shocked and moved by the tragic and horrific death of Baby P. All of us find it impossible to comprehend how adults could commit such terrible acts of evil against this little boy. And the public is angry that nobody stepped in to prevent this tragedy from happening . . . Nothing we do now can take away the terrible suffering that was inflicted on Baby P during his short life. (Balls 2008)

Balls announced that he had initiated a series of inquiries into child protection in Haringey by Ofsted, The Health Care Commission and the Chief Inspector of Constabulary. He blamed Haringey Council, especially its Director of Social Services, for the disaster and ordered the Council to immediately remove her from her post and replace her with his nominee, and asked Ofsted to review the progress of the Council in implementing the recommendation of the inspectors. Ed Balls ended his statement: 'We will not rest until we have the very best child protection arrangements in Haringey and across our country' (2008).

While ministers tend to make public statements about policy or failings, they are supported by civil servants, especially departmental press officers (usually former journalists), who seek to promote positive images of the Minister and his or her actions and counteract negative images. To facilitate this, the press officers, popularly known as spin doctors, seek to develop close informal relations with the national media. Former ministers have been critical of the influence of media officers in the policy process. For example, Clare Short, who was the Minister responsible for International Development (1997–2003), described the relationship in the following way:

> Spin degrades journalism as well as politics. Spin works because journalists queue up for briefings from those who are seen to be close to power. They are kept in line with leaks, prior announcements and background briefings. Those who refuse to toe the line are deprived of access. Spin meisters enhance their power by demonstrating their 'control' of the media. Their advice is taken before policy is decided. Through background briefing they puff or weaken politicians and thus extend their influence. (Short cited in Katwala, Whitford and Ottery 2003)

When governments wish to conceal issues, they may issue information in ways that do not attract media attention. For example, in 1980 the Conservative Government wanted to distance itself from the Report of the Working Party on Inequalities (the Black Report) established by the preceding Labour Government. Instead of using Her Majesty's Stationery Office to publish the report, the Department of Health and Social Security issued 260 duplicated copies on an August Bank Holiday (Townsend and Davidson 1982: 11). A more extreme approach to burying bad news can be seen in the memorandum which Jo Moore, a press officer at the Department of Transport, sent to her colleagues on 11 September 2001 after the attack on the World Trade Center in New York, suggesting it was a good day to bury bad news. She and her boss, Martin Sixsmith, resigned in February 2002 following a row over another memorandum in which she suggested that the department should release poor rail performance figures on the day of Princess Margaret's funeral (*BBC News* 2002; Sparrow 2001).

These government strategies to influence the ways in which the media represent their policies have been undermined by the changing nature of the media. New technology has facilitated greater competition between media outlets and increased the speed of media response to events – for example, 24-hour news programmes, plus regularly up-dated on-line websites, mean that the media comments on events virtually as they happen. As Kavanagh and his colleagues note: 'A by-product of more continuous, intensive and competitive coverage of politics seems to have led to more concentration on crises, scandals, personal rivalries and division' (2006: 511). At the same time as politics has become more personalised and critical, ministers and civil servants have less time to anticipate and respond to issues and criticisms raised by the media.

The trend to focus on the personal failings of policy makers has been reinforced by broader social change that is reflected in and reinforced by the mass media. As we noted earlier in this chapter, modern journalism developed a distinctive matrix combining generalised abstract 'facts' with personal accounts of natural disasters, such as the 1665 London Plague and the 1755 Lisbon earthquake. A new element has been added to the matrix – personal responsibility or blame. Increasingly, disasters are presented as man-made rather than natural. As we noted in chapter 5, modern society is increasingly dominated by a blame culture.

Given the increased scope of government responsibility, its actions and policies are subject to mass media scrutiny especially in the contexts of disasters. It is possible to identify a sequence of media and government interactions in such situations:

• *Initial identification of disaster* As we noted in chapter 5, the media identify some events as shocking, i.e. threatening to the normal established order of everyday life. The shock involves an emotional or horror element which may reflect the level of harm, such as the number of deaths and injuries. But as we noted in the discussion of media coverage of Mods and Rockers, high levels of harm are not necessary for events to be constructed as shocking and a threat. As a former Prime Minister noted in his analysis of the media, increased competitiveness means that individual media outlets seek to make an impact and 'The audience needs to be arrested, held and their emotions engaged. Something that is interesting is less powerful than something that makes you angry or shocked' (Blair 2007: 4). Part of this impact involves scrutinising the reaction of government officials who are expected to empathise with the victims and take immediate action to ameliorate their situation.

- *Media frenzy* When events become generally accepted as a disaster and all mass media outlets focus on the events, they become front-page news in the newspapers and lead stories on the TV news. Alongside images and coverage of the harm and victims, there is increased analysis of the causes of the disaster – especially societal and governmental failings. This search for those who are responsible and whose lack of foresight contributed to the disaster results in a media frenzy, 'the fear of missing out means today's media, more than ever before, hunts in a pack. In these modes it is like a feral beast, just tearing people and reputations to bits. But no-one dares miss out' (Blair 2007: 5).

- *Pressure for immediate reaction and action* As Blair indicated, the development of a more fragmented media with rapid on-line production has reduced the time policy makers have to respond to issues. He noted how in the 1960s the government could have a two-day cabinet meeting to reflect on an important issue, while at the time of writing 'It would be laughable to think you could do that now without the heavens falling in before lunch on the first day' (2007: 3). As a result there is no time for rational reflection as policy makers virtually have to access relevant evidence as they are giving it to the media. There is pressure for immediate action. In the case of the Mods and Rockers moral panic in 1964, the Government's immediate response was to present a planned policy change as if it was a response to the threat of the Mods and Rockers (the 1964 Drugs (Prevention of Misuse) Act) and to introduce new legislation designed to deal with the vandalism associated with the Mods and Rockers, the 1964 Malicious Damage Act (Cohen 2002: 110–15). Media coverage of the harm caused by dangerous dogs also resulted in 'knee jerk' policy making. From 1989 to 1991 the tabloid media carried reports and images of children attacked by dogs, and the Home Secretary had stonewalled media demands for action (Lodge and Hood 2002: 6). However, on the weekend of the 18–19 May 1991, there was extensive media coverage of the case of a six-year-old from Bradford who was attacked. On 21 May, the Prime Minister referred in Parliament to the horrific attack and announced that the Government would take action. The following day, Home Secretary Kenneth Baker introduced a bill to ban four types of dangerous dogs, including pit bull terriers, and the Dangerous Dogs Act became law on 12 August 1991 (Parkinson 2009). This Act was neither instrumentally rational, i.e. there was no evidence that it reduced the incidence of dog attacks, especially on children (Parkinson 2009; Klaasen, Buckley and Esmail 1996) – nor communicatively rational – the tabloid newspapers which had called for tough government action were soon 'carrying tear-jerking stories' of much-loved family pets condemned to death (Lodge and Hood 2002: 6).

Comment

Though policy makers would like to have the time and space to reflect on the best way to respond to issues, the development of fragmented competitive mass media looking for quick solutions and ready to allocate blame creates pressure for immediate action. Thus policy makers can be seen as reacting to the agenda being set by the mass media and having to make rapid decisions in the spotlight of media attention (see table 9.1 for a comparison of rational and media-driven policy making).

Table 9.1   Rational versus media-driven policy making

	Policy making grounded in instrumental rationality	Media-driven policy making
Role of policy makers	Proactive, predicting and managing the future	Reactive, especially to the current crisis
Pressure/time	Time for reflection	Need for rapid response
Focus	Broad focus on creating a better future	Narrow response to immediate issues
Forum	A degree of insulation from external pressure	Highly visible and public, no insulation or barriers
Emotion	Mechanisms to screen out affect	Central, need to show concern
Blame	Not a key issue	A central concern for policy makers

KEY POINTS

- *Modernity and mediated representation* With the move from intimate small-scale local communities to impersonal large-scale urban societies, individuals can no longer rely on direct personal experience as their prime source of knowledge, but use mediated representations to access knowledge about distant events that may have important effects upon their lives.
- *Development of journalism and the narrative matrix* Mediated representations are made convincing through a combination of authoritativeness – i.e. factual evidence and scientific explanation – and authenticity – i.e. personal eye witness accounts.
- *Mass media templates* Given that each event is unique, to make it understandable to a potential audience the mass media use templates in which previous iconic events 'explain' the new event by providing a link with a known and pre-existing group of events or anchor.
- *Accountability, blame and the narrative matrix* With the increasing emphasis on the man-made rather than the natural components of disasters, the explanatory component in the narrative matrix has expanded to include not only natural scientific explanations but also social and human factors. Such explanations facilitate the allocation of blame to specific individuals.
- *Media-driven policy making* The development of a proactive mass media actively looking for scandals and disasters places considerable pressure on policy makers. It limits the scope for rational planning and creates a personalised and emotive environment in which policy makers are expected to empathise, show sincerity, take immediate action – including punishing those who failed in their allocated tasks – and make policies that will prevent such disasters happening again.

Part 3
Conclusion

10

So how and why are health policies made? Some final comments

AIMS

- To examine the various factors which impinge on and shape the ways in which health policy is made in the UK.

OBJECTIVES

- To consider the importance of instrumental rationality as both the justification of and reality of heath policy making
- To explore the factors that limit the scope of instrumental rationality.

In this concluding chapter we reflect on the ways in which health policy has been and is made. We note the ways in which core policy makers seek to make rational policy and we note the challenges that they face. We reflect on the ways in which policy making is context-specific with rational elements being evident in some contexts but other factors predominating in most.

10.1 Policy makers and the changing environment of policy making

In modern democracies policy makers' accounts of policy making emphasise the role of instrumental rationality. In such accounts policy makers act altruistically to identify major social issues and to make decisions which create a better future for all citizens. The instrumental rationality of policy making justifies the status and power of policy makers: they are not acting in their own interest but in the public interest and for the public good. Policy makers are striving for the best possible future for society, one which is efficient – i.e. maximises the use of resources; effective – maximises out-puts of benefits; and just – allocating benefits according to agreed criteria such as need. Instrumental rationality with its straightforward assumptions regarding the appropriateness of certain ends, alongside the evaluation and selection of optimum means to these ends, provides a clear basis for such a future.

In the United Kingdom core policy makers – ministers and their confidential advisers (especially civil servants) – enjoy high status and considerable power. The United Kingdom is a highly central-ised state which has been referred to as an 'elective dictatorship' (Hailsham 1976), in which ministers have taken over the powers and some of the ceremony of a medieval monarchy. The ability of the British Prime Minister and his or her ministers to develop and implement new policies tends to exceed that of the US President and his ministers, who are forced to negotiate and compromise with an often hostile Congress. For example, in the last twenty years or so the British government has undertaken repeated restructuring of the system of health care – for example, *Working for Patients* (Department of Health 1989) and *New NHS: Modern, Dependable* (Department of Health 1997); in the USA plans to reform health care either failed (Clinton's 1993 health-care plan) or were diluted (Obama's 2010 health-care reforms).

Although the policy-making core in the UK retains much of its authority, it has also experienced a crisis of confidence, and policy makers perceive themselves as working in a relatively hostile envi-ronment in which they are increasingly called upon to account for their actions. At the start of the twentieth century, a small elite of policy makers in Whitehall made policy not only for the UK and its emerging welfare system but also for a global empire. This small elite worked in a club culture in which shared generalist education (elite public schools) and common implicit values (muscular Christianity and a strong sense of British superiority) formed the basis for a system oriented to minimising overt public conflict through a system of tacit rules, close face-to-face relations and mutual respect and trust. Difficulties were sorted out in private through compromises made behind closed doors.

Key elements of this system survived well into the late twentieth century. In the 1950s the relationship between civil servants and officials of the BMA was based on first-name terms and involved private face-to-face 'backstairs' discussions and negotiations on all aspects of health policy, including the minutiae of health service administration (Eckstein 1960). Similarly in the 1960s, key public expenditure decisions were made in the 'Whitehall Village' and civil servants prioritised maintaining mutually beneficial relations and the consensus over making the best allocation decisions (Heclo and Wildavsky 1981: l).

Some elements of early-twentieth-century government have survived into the twenty-first century. Following the May 2010 general election, a small elite of policy makers in Whitehall still controlled policy making, though the focus was on economic and welfare policy in the UK not on sustaining a global empire. This elite had changed in some ways: it was now more middle- than upper-class, and included (some) women and individuals from ethnic minority backgrounds, and more diversity of education. While elite public school and university education was still prominent, there was increasing emphasis on specialist knowledge and expertise and less evidence of shared values. For example, in the negotiations following the 2010 election the parties had to articulate and reach a compromise over their key values – electoral reform in the case of the Liberal Democrats and reduction of public expenditure and the state in the case of the Conservatives. There was also an important change to the normal process of transferring power from one government and party to the next in which, following an election, one Prime Minister immediately resigns to be replaced by the next. Following the 2010 election, the Prime Minister, Gordon Brown, did not resign but retained office until negotiations over the formation of the next government were nearly complete. Although these negotiations marked a departure from the normal smooth transfer of power, in other ways they followed UK precedent. They took place behind closed doors and there was enough mutual respect and trust for the negotiators from each party to reach agreement on key issues (Iannucci 2010).

Though the negotiations took place in private, the key participants defended their decisions to their political parties, to Parliament, and through the media, to the public. While the Coalition had the basic requirements for the formation of a government – a working majority in the House of Commons – its partners felt the need to stress the popular support of such a government. This self-consciousness reflected not just the unusual conditions of a coalition government and the challenges of managing a continuing economic crisis including tax increases and reductions in welfare benefits, but also an underlying concern about legitimacy. Iannucci, in commenting on the 'behind-closed-doors' coalition negotiations argued that: 'Over the past 15 years or so, the electorate has become increasingly disaffected by and disengaged from the political process, at the same time as the political classes have claimed to be acting more and more in response to our opinions' (2010: 23).

The erosion of the self-confidence of core policy makers and their increased need for popular support and endorsement can be traced back to the economic and political crises of the 1970s. These crises represented a major challenge to the traditional ways of making policy, especially those which formed part of the traditional Whitehall club culture. The financial crisis of 1974/6 during which the Treasury effectively lost control of public expenditure indicated the limits of a system in which maintaining relations was prioritised over policy outcomes. The crisis coincided with, and created the opportunity for, the election of radical governments with strong ideologically grounded programmes of reform. Such governments were hostile to a system oriented to stability and the maintenance of established relations.

In the case of the Labour Government (1974–9) with its socialist orientation, a move towards a more corporatist system of policy making meant that the Government was more receptive to claims from the trade unions and others that challenged the privileges of the established elites, e.g. the access which medical practitioners had to pay beds within NHS hospitals. The radical Conservative Government, elected in 1979 and influenced by the New Right ideologies, treated the medical profession as another self-interested group seeking to sustain expenditure on welfare and proceeded to make major policies (*Working for Patients*: Department of Health 1989) without the involvement of the profession, thus breaking up the traditional club culture of health policy making.

The crisis of the 1970s reflected broader changes in society that made the environment of policy making more challenging and made it more difficult for policy makers to carry on making policy behind closed doors. These included:

• *Increased incidence and impact of disasters* Disasters are clear evidence that current policies have failed and that policy makers are at fault. Policy makers can appoint inquiries to deflect blame and defuse the emotional tensions which build up around the disaster. Indeed some ministers, such as Richard Crossman in the late 1960s and Alan Milburn in the late 1990s, used disasters to justify their programmes of reform and change. However, inquiries force policy making into the public arena. Inquiries usually make public the evidence they collect, their analysis of the causes of the disaster, the individuals they find to be at fault and their recommendations for policy changes to prevent a repetition of the disaster. Ministers are forced to publicly respond to these recommendations and to accept them unless they can find compelling reasons not to.

- *More aggressive and critical media* Since the 1960s there has been development of new media, such as the internet, and increased competition between existing media, such as the tabloid press. Although policy makers, especially spin doctors, seek to control this more aggressive media, given the newsworthiness of disasters and scandals, policy makers are often forced to respond rapidly to events. Such rapid responses limit the scope for rational planning and create a personalised and emotive environment in which policy makers are expected to respond to disasters by empathising with the victims, taking immediate action, including punishing those who failed in their allocated tasks, and making policies that will prevent disasters happening again.

- *Development of a risk and blaming culture* Traditional political ideologies such as socialism, have been replaced with newer ones such as New Labour's Third Way. At one level this is a pragmatic fusion of earlier ideologies, but at another it builds on new concepts such as risk and choice. Risk can be seen as a neutral technology for predicting and managing the future and therefore as a way of protecting people and enhancing their safety. In this sense, it fits into the instrumental rational model of policy making, providing a way of controlling the future and maximising social benefit in terms of minimising harm. However, risk becomes a double-edged sword when used forensically and applied to the past. The concept of risk can and is used in the same way as sin is in religious societies – to identify (moral) failing and to allocate blame in the context of disasters (Douglas 1990). This underpins the development of a 'blame culture', in which all harmful events are seen as a product of human agency and every misfortune is someone's fault: 'under the banner of risk reduction, a new blaming system has replaced the former' system based on religion and sin (Douglas 1992: 16). If the media succeed in identifying the 'guilty' party, then a disaster becomes a scandal and there is pressure for the guilty to be punished. Since policy makers claim to provide safe health and social care, they must find ways of deflecting blame when things go wrong – as they increasingly do in such health and social care systems which are tightly coupled with little slack (Perrow 1999: 4).

- *Increased power of sevice users* Governments in the early twenty-first century are committed to increasing user participation in health policy making and service delivery. This means that policy makers need to show that they are responsive to and value consumer and public views. As we noted in chapter 4, in the run-up to the 2001 election, when Health Ministers decided to issue a major policy statement, *The NHS Plan* (Department of Health 2000a), they based it on a review of public attitudes and opinion. Similarly Darzi (2007) justified his proposals for the restructuring of the NHS in London in terms of public support: 'we have based the *Framework* on what Londoners have told us they want, so I believe we will have the public's support for the proposed changes' (pp. 2–3). The increasing importance of consumers and their representation means that policy makers have to open policy making to increase public participation. Policy makers have accepted that public confidence and the trust of citizens are central to public services – in the case of the NHS through ensuring it is a 'high trust' organisation (Department of Health 2000b: 56).

10.2 The changing nature of the health policy process

Consensus and prosperity: the simplicity of policy making in the early years of the NHS

In the late 1940s and 1950s the health and social care policy system was relatively simple, with participation limited mainly to insiders and its outcomes relatively predictable. The Ministry of Health was at the centre of a policy community which included officials of the BMA and relevant civil servants in the Treasury. The main focus of this community was the effective delivery of health and social care through services administered by the NHS and local authorities, and for the most part its policy making fell within the area of low politics, routine issues which did not threaten the continued existence of the government. Those issues which did become matters of high politics were the ones that the policy community did not have the capacity to deal with: doctors' pay and the overall costs of the NHS where the BMA was constrained by its membership and the Ministry of Health by the Treasury.

In many ways this system worked well. In the 1950s health and social-care systems operated with high public support, little evidence of poor-quality care and few complaints. For members of the policy community it was a highly rational system. It operated at low cost, served the interests of its members, was mutually beneficial and provided for stable long-term relationships. Outside the policy community there was little intrusion into or interest in the policy-making process from other potential participants such as political parties, parliament, pressure groups, the media or the public. Thus, when Enoch Powell announced the Hospital Plan in 1962 there had been little public debate or involvement in the process, and media coverage focused on the level of public investment with little discussion of the importance of the new district general hospitals for the overall pattern of health and social services and their implications for patients such as increased travel time.

Health policy making in the twenty-first century

Since the 1950s health policy making has substantially increased in scope and complexity. In some areas rational instrumentality and professional expertise still play a key role.

In the 1950s the policy community did not explicitly deal with the issue of clinical standards. This was a matter for professional self-regulation, and the various Royal Colleges played a key role with their approval of training facilities and training posts. With the development of clinical governance in 1997, ministers and the Department of Health needed clinical standards against which they could assess the quality and performance of services and clinicians. The Government drew on professional expertise through the appointment of National Clinical Directors or 'Tsars' for the specific disease groups or service areas. These Directors are tasked with developing policy within their clinical areas by ensuring that expert groups collect and codify the best-quality clinical evidence, and this evidence informs National Service Frameworks – evidence-based strategies which 'set clear requirements for care' (National Health Service 2010) for each client or disease area. The Directors are responsible for ensuring that these Frameworks or their equivalent form the basis for the development of local services and are supported by implementation teams within the Department.

However even these supposedly rational parts of the policy-making system are not totally insulated from external pressure. While expert working parties remain an important part of the process of developing Frameworks, they are complemented by a new organisation, the National Institute for Health and Clinical Excellence (NICE). This is an 'arm's-length' organisation, funded by the Government but operating independently. Its role is to develop an overall evidence base of encoded scientific knowledge for the NHS. It uses technical expertise, often from university research units, to access and summarise the evidence on current practice, provide guidance on current best practice and to evaluate the benefit of existing and new forms of treatment. NICE uses QALYs (Quality Adjusted Life Years) as the basis of its rational judgement of whether a treatment should be routinely funded by the NHS. If the treatment costs less than £20,000 per QALY then the intervention is considered to be cost-effective. If a QALY costs between £20,000 and £30,000, then the treatment is only beneficial if there are other intangible benefits. Generally a treatment that costs more than £30,000 per QALY is not considered beneficial (NICE 2008: 19).

While this all appears very technical and rational, the actual decision making is often more complex and contested. We noted that NICE reviewed Herceptin, a drug that reduced the mortality of women who have an aggressive HER2 form of breast cancer. The review of evidence found that Herceptin did reduce mortality and that each QALY cost £14,069; however, when the side-effects of treatment were factored in, this cost rose to £29,448. Although Herceptin was on the margin of cost-effectiveness, NICE decided to recommend its approval. When this decision is examined in more detail it is clear that contingent factors, i.e. those outside the review of evidence, played an important role. While Herceptin was under review, groups representing women who had had breast cancer and the pharmaceutical company that developed the drug mounted a high-profile media campaign stressing the 'other factors' that should be considered, i.e. despite the cost of the Herceptin, there was no other drug that was effective in reducing the mortality of HER2 breast cancer.

NICE's decision over the use of Beta interferon to treat a form of multiple sclerosis was also subject to external pressures. In 2000 NICE completed its review of evidence that indicated that Beta interferon was not cost-effective, but before it could announce its decision it was leaked to the media. An informal alliance of user groups, medical specialists and pharmaceutical companies forced NICE to defer its decision and commission a further review. This confirmed the initial judgement not to recommend the use of Beta interferon. However, at the same time the Government effectively by-passed NICE and negotiated a compromise deal with the drug manufacturers that reduced the cost of the drug to the NHS, facilitating the treatment of about one in six MS patients.

Contingency and policy making

While policy decisions about treatment guidelines and the cost-effectiveness of treatment regimes may approximate to instrumental rationality, in other areas of health and social-care policy-making rationality tends to be overwhelmed by contingent factors. This is perhaps most evident when considering the identification of the ends of policy. While the ends or outcomes which rational policy is designed to achieve should be a key issue, in practice most descriptions and prescriptions of rational policy making focus on evaluation of means – the ends of policy tend to be taken as self-evident or as a given. It is relatively easy to assume that the purpose of health policy is to improve health or to reduce mortality; the difficulties begin to emerge when these issues are defined more closely. Perhaps the only model of rational policy making to address the issue of the ends that policy should be addressing is the mixed scanning approach that involves scanning of the future to identify emerging issues that are likely to become policy problems. It is possible to identify such future scanning in the Treasury-commissioned review of the NHS. Sir Derek Wanless (2002) was invited to review the long-term cost trends of health care in the United Kingdom. The review was supported by the Health Trends Review team in the Treasury and also commissioned research on the health trends and costs in eight other countries. The review identified two crucial issues which would affect the cost and development of the NHS: the public take-up of public health advice, and willingness of NHS managers and clinicians to use health-care resources efficiently.

However, such a rational approach to the identification of issues is exceptional. Key policy issues tend to emerge from two sources, disasters and claims-makers, and both these sources contribute to the modern narrative matrix of the mass media – mixing facts, emotions and morality. The contribution of these contingent factors is clearly evident in the reform of mental health legislation. The disasters of the 1990s, such as the killing of Jonathan Zito by Christopher Clunis, resulted in a series of inquiries that emphasised the threat posed by people with mental illness, recommended the use of risk techniques to identify and manage this dangerousness and became media templates for mental illness that reinforced public perceptions of the dangerousness of people with mental illness. In 1997, Frank

Dobson, the new Secretary of State for Health, influenced by the New Labour risk and blame ideology accepted media representation of the dangerousness of people with mental illness, the failure of voluntary treatment of people with mental illness in the community, and the need for compulsory treatment in the community of those individuals who would not cooperate.

In the rational model there is a clear separation between the identification of policy aims and the process of evaluating the best means of achieving such ends. In the case of the Review of the future costs of the NHS, Wanless (2002) identified the key issues, but a consideration of the best way of managing these issues was beyond the scope of the Review. However, in reality, ends and means are rarely clearly separated and they are entangled in the policy process. This entanglement was clear in the case of mental health policy. Dobson clearly identified the ends of policy – more effective management of the risks from people with mental illness – and also the best way of achieving this, compulsory treatment in the community. Even though the Government had a large majority in the House of Commons and the new policy was relatively low-cost as it mainly involved new legislation to introduce Community Treatment Orders, the reform of the law was delayed for some ten years (Mental Health Act 2007) and, although it did extend compulsory treatment to the patients in the community, the Act took the form of an amendment of an earlier Act (1983 Mental Health Act), rather than a completely new review and statement of the law. Dobson was opposed by an alliance of mental health clinicians and representatives of users of services who challenged his definition of the problem. They claimed that there was no evidence that people with mental illness had become any more dangerous or a serious threat to public safety. They claimed that people with mental illness were more likely to be the victims of neglect and stigma than the perpetrators of violence. Thus they argued that policy should be addressing a different problem – namely, how to identify and meet the needs of people with mental illness. This problem would not be addressed by increased legal powers but required additional funding of services. The effectiveness of such counterclaims in initially delaying and subsequently shaping both the definition of the problem and its solution reflects both the effectiveness of the alliance in organising opposition and the key veto power of the Royal College of Psychiatrists.

Contingent factors make policy making both more unpredictable and more interesting. Instrumental rationality aims to simplify and manage an unpredictable future to maximise social benefits.

Where such rationality can be identified, as in some elements of public expenditure and in the role of Clinical Directors and NICE, policy making becomes a highly technical exercise which involves the almost mechanical accumulation and analysis of evidence. In contrast, events such as disasters, pressure groups making claims about the problems that government should deal with and the media making moral judgements about the failure of policy makers all add to the unpredictability and excitement of policy making and emphasise the limits of instrumentality.

Comment

It is possible to identify some of the factors that influence the outcome of policy making. For example, groups with veto power, the most resources, that are the most media-savvy and/or have good evidence to support their claims are likely to have the greatest influence on policy outcomes. However, the outcome depends on circumstances. In the case of the 1996 Dunblane killings, a small group with minimal resources, no experience of working with the media or strong evidence to support their claim that handguns were intrinsically dangerous took on the gun lobby, made up of well-funded groups, with considerable media expertise, close relationships to the policy-making core and good evidence to support their claims that it was the person using the gun, rather than the gun itself which posed the danger. In this case public, media and political support meant that David defeated Goliath.

KEY POINTS

- In the United Kingdom core policy makers enjoy high status and considerable power. They have the capacity to identify policy problems, determine the best solutions and take actions to implement such solutions.
- Although the policy-making core in the UK retains much of its authority, it has also experienced a crisis of confidence, and policy makers perceive themselves as working in a relatively hostile environment in which they are increasingly called upon to account for their actions.
- Policy makers aspire to rational instrumental policy making, and in some areas of health policy it is possible to identify such policy making.

- However, such rational approaches to the identification of issues are exceptional. Key policy issues tend to emerge from two sources, disasters and claims-makers, and both these sources contribute to the modern narrative matrix of the mass media that mixes facts, emotions and morality.

References

Aberfan (n.d.) The Aberfan disaster, http://www.nuffield.ox.ac.uk/politics/
aberfan/home2.htmin, accessed 13 July 2007.

Abraham, J. (2009) The pharmaceutical industry, the state and the NHS.
In *The New Sociology of the Health Service*, ed. J. Gabe and M. Calnan.
London: Routledge, pp. 99–120.

Adorno, T. and Horkheimer, M. (1972) *Dialectic of Enlightenment*. London:
Verso.

Alaszewski, A. (1983) The development of policy for the mentally handicapped since the Second World War: an introduction. *Oxford Review of
Education*. 9: 227–31.

Alaszewski, A. (2002) The impact of the Bristol Royal Infirmary disaster and
inquiry on public services in the UK. *Journal of Interprofessional Care*. 16
(4): 371–78.

Alaszewski, A. (2003) Risk, clinical governance and best value: restoring
confidence in health and social care. In *Clinical Governance and Best Value:
Meeting the Modernization Agenda*, ed. S. Pickering and J. Thompson.
Edinburgh: Churchill Livingstone, pp.171–82.

Alaszewski, A. (2011) How campaigners and the media push bad science.
BMJ 342: d236, http://www.bmj.com/content/342/bmj.d236.full,
accessed 21 April 2011.

Alaszewski, A. and Brown, P. (2007) Risk, uncertainty and knowledge.
Health, Risk and Society. 9(1): 1–10.

Alaszewski, A. and Burgess, A. (2007) Risk, time and reason. *Health, Risk
and Society*. 9 (4): 349–58.

Alaszewski, A. and Coxon, K. (2008) The everyday experience of living with
risk and uncertainty. *Health, Risk and Society*. 10 (5): 413–20.

Alford, R.R. (1975) *Health Care Politics: Ideological and Interest Group Barriers
to Reform*. Chicago: University of Chicago Press.

Allen, D.E. (1979) *Hospital Planning: The Development of the 1962 Hospital
Plan*. London: Pitman Medical.

Allen, G. (2003) *The Last Prime Minister: Being Honest about the UK Presidency*. Thorverton: Imprint Academic.

Appleby, J. and Dixon, J. (2004) Patient choice in the NHS: having choice may not improve health outcomes. *BMJ*. 329: 61–2.

Archer, M. (1998) Introduction. In *Critical Realism: Essential readings*, ed. M. Archer, R. Bhaskar, A. Collier, T. Lawson and A. Norrie. London: Routledge, pp ix–xiv.

Baggott, R. (2005) A funny thing happened on the way to the forum? Reforming patient and public involvement in the NHS in England. *Public Administration*. 83 (3): 533–51.

Baker, M. (2000) *Making Sense of the NHS White Papers*. 2nd edition. Abingdon: Radcliffe Medical Press.

Baker, R. (n.d.) Public health-biographies. Report on the Sanitary Condition of the Labouring Population. http://www.bl.uk/learning/histcitizen/21cc/publichealth/background/biographies/publichealthbiographies.html, accessed 21 June 2010.

Balls, E. (2008) Baby P: Ed Balls' statement in full. http://www.guardian.co.uk/society/2008/dec/01/baby-p-ed-balls-statement. accessed 9 April 2010.

Barker, R. and Storey, C. (1992) Coping without Crown immunity in the NHS. *Health and Safety at Work*. 14: 37–8.

Barnes, C. (1992) *Disabling Imagery and the Media: An Exploration of the Principles for Media Representations of Disabled People*. Krumlin: The British Council of Organizations of Disabled People and Ryburn Publishing.

BBC (2005) Call to reform mental health plan. http://news.bbc.co.uk/1/hi/health/4372821.stm, accessed 10 August 2005.

BBC News (1997) Blair apologies for mishandling F1 row. *BBC News* 17 November 1997. http://news.bbc.co.uk/1/hi/uk/31780.stm, accessed 9 April 2010.

BBC News (1999) Health: 'Acceptable mistakes' at scandal hospital. *BBC News* 11 November 1999. http://news.bbc.co.uk/1/hi/health/515733.stm. accessed 20 April 2010.

BBC News (2000) Dorrell regrets BSE statement. *BBC News* 27 October 2000. http://news.bbc.co/1/hi/uk/993757.stm, accessed 21 March 2010.

BBC News (2002) Spin memo row duo quit. *BBC News* 15 February 2002. http://news.bbc.co.uk/1/hi/uk_politics/1823120.stm. accessed 8 April 2010.

BBC News (2008) 1957 Britons 'have never had it so good'. On this day, 1950–2005, 20 July. http://news.bbc.co.uk/onthisday/hi/dates/stories/july/20/newsid_3728000/3728225.stm, accessed 13 April 2011.

Beattie, J. (1966) *Other Cultures: Aims, Methods and Achievements in Social Anthropology*. London: Routledge and Kegan Paul.

Beck, U. (1992) *Risk Society: Towards a New Modernity*. London: Sage.

Beharrell, P. (1993) AIDS and the British press. In *Getting the Message: News, Truth and Power*, ed. J. Eldridge. London and New York: Routledge, pp. 210–49.

Bell, D. (1960) *The End of Ideology: On the Exhaustion of Political Ideas in the Fifties*. Cambridge, Mass.: Harvard University Press.

Bentham, J. (1977) [1776] *A Comment on the Commentaries and A Fragment on Government*. Reprint edited by J. H. Burns and H. L. A. Hart. London: The Athlone Press.

Bentham, J. (2000) [1781] *An Introduction to the Principles of Morals and Legislation*. http://socserv.mcmaster.ca/econ/ugcm/3113/bentham/morals. pdf, accessed 1 October 2009.

Berger, P. and Luckmann, T. (1966) *The Social Construction of Reality*. London: Penguin.

Bernard, M. and Phillips, J. (2000) The challenge of ageing in tomorrow's Britain. *Ageing and Society*. 20: 33–54.

Best, J. (1995) Typification and social problem construction. In *Images of Issues: Typifying Contemporary Social Problems*, ed. J. Best. New York: Aldine De Gruyter, pp 1–16.

Best, J. (1999) *Random Violence: How We Talk about New Crimes and New Victims*. Berkeley: University of California Press.

Best, J. and Loseke, D. (2003) *Social Problems: Constructionist Readings*. New York: Aldine de Gruyter.

Beveridge, W. (1942) *Social Insurance and Allied Services: Report by Sir William Beveridge*. Cmd 6404. London: HMSO.

Blair, T. (1998) Foreword. In *Modern Public Services for Britain: Investing in Reform: Comprehensive Spending Review: New Public Spending Plans 1999–2002, July 1998*. http://www.archive.official-documents.co.uk/document/ cm40/4011/foreword.htm, accessed 13 August 2009.

Blair, T. (1999) Foreword. In *Modernising Government*. Cm 4310. London. TSO. http://www.archive.official-documents.co.uk/document/ cm43/4310/4310-fw.htm, accessed 11 June 2010.

Blair, T. (2007) Lecture by the Prime Minister on Public Life, Reuters, Canary Wharf, London, Tuesday 12 June 2007. http://image.guardian. co.uk/sys-files/Politics/documents/2007/06/12/BlairReuterSpeech.pdf, accessed 12 April 2010.

Blaxter, M. and Paterson, E. (1982) *Mothers and Daughters: A Three-generational Study of Health Attitudes and Behaviour*. London: Heinemann Educational Books.

Blom-Cooper, L. (1996) Some reflections on public inquiries. In *Inquiries after homicide*, ed. J. Peay. London: Duckworth.

Braybrooke , D. and Lindblom, C. E. (1963) *A Strategy of Decision*. New York: Free Press.

Bristol Royal Infirmary Inquiry (2001) *Learning from Bristol, The Report of the Public Inquiry into Children's Heart Surgery at the Bristol Royal Infirmary 1984–1995*, Chair Ian Kennedy, Cm 5207, http://www.bristol-inquiry. org.uk/, accessed 12 July 2007 and 27 April 2010.

Bröer, C. (2007) Aircraft noise and risk politics. *Health, Risk and Society*. 9 (1): 37–52.

Brown, C. and Morris, N. (2007) Brown completes government of 'all talents' with team of outsiders. *Independent*, 30 June 2007. http://www. independent.co.uk/news/uk/politics/brown-completes-government-of-all-talents-with-team-of-outsiders-455341.html, accessed 14 April 2011.

Brown, R. G. S. and Steel, D. R. (1979) *The Administrative Process in Britain*. 2nd edition. London: Methuen.

Brown, P. (2006). Risk versus need in revising the 1983 Mental Health Act: conflicting claims, muddled policy. *Health, Risk and Society*. 8 (4): 343–58.

Brown, P. (2008a) Trusting in the new NHS: instrumental *versus* communicative action. *Sociology of Health and Illness*. 30 (3): 349–63.

Brown, P. (2008b) Legitimacy chasing its own tail: theorising clinical governance through a critique of instrumental reason. *Social Theory and Health*. 6: 184–99.

Brown, P. and Calnan, M. (2010) The risks of managing uncertainty: the limitations of governance and choice, and the potential for trust. *Social Policy and Society*. 9 (1).

Brown, P. and Flores, R. (2011) Making normative structures visible: the British National Health Service and the hospice movement as signifiers of compassion and hope. *Acta Sociologica*. 54 (1): 61–75.

BSE Inquiry (2001) *The Report*, Vol. I: *Findings and Conclusions. The Inquiry into BSE and variant CJD in the United Kingdom*. http://web.archive.org/web/20001109072700/www.bseinquiry.gov.uk/report/volume1/toc.htm, accessed 18 June 2010.

Burchell, G., Gordon, C. and Miller. P. (eds.)(1991) *The Foucault Effect – Studies in Governmentality*. Hemel Hempstead: Harvester Wheatsheaf.

Burgess, A. (2004) *Cellular Phones, Public Fears and a Culture of Precaution*. New York: Cambridge University Press.

Burgess, A. (2009) Commentary: the politics of health risk promotion. 'Passive drinking': a 'good lie' too far? *Health, Risk and Society*. 11: 527–40.

Butler, I. and Drakeford, M. (2005) *Scandal, Social Policy and Social Welfare*. 2nd edition. Basingstoke: Palgrave Macmillan.

Cabinet Office (2008) *List of Ministerial Responsibilities Including Executive Agencies and Non-Ministerial Departments*. London: Cabinet Office. http://lmr.cabinetoffice.gov.uk/media/4506/lmr_november2008.pdf, accessed 1 December 2008.

Cabinet Office (2011a) *Big Society – overview*, http://www.cabinetoffice.gov. uk/content/big-society-overview, accessed 14 April 2011.

Cabinet Office (2011b) *Building a new culture of social responsibility*, http://www. cabinetoffice.gov.uk/news/building-new-culture-social-responsibility, accessed 14 April 2011.

Calman, K. and Hine, D. (1995) *A Policy Framework for Commissioning Cancer Services: A Report by the Expert Advisory Group on Cancer to the Chief Medical Officers of England and Wales*. London: Department of Health.

Campos, P. (2004) *The Obesity Myth: Why America's Obsession with Weight is Hazardous to your Health*. New York: Gotham Books.

Carson, R. (1962) *Silent Spring*. London: Hamish Hamilton.

Carvel, J. (2007) Trust failed to warn of outbreak or improve hygiene. http://www.guardian.co.uk/society/2007/oct/11/health1, accessed 24 April 2010.

Castle, B. (1980) *The Castle Diaries 1974–76*. London: George Weidenfeld and Nicolson.

Cawson, A. (1986) *Corporatism and Political Theory*. Oxford: Basil Blackwell.

Chapman, R.A. (1997) *The Treasury in Public Policy-making*. London: Routledge.

CIPFA (2007) *Zero Based Budgeting*, http://www.cipfa.org.uk/pt/download/zero_based_budgeting_briefing.pdf, accessed 29 July 2009.

Clarke, N. (2007) Cover-ups, lies and the cynical conspiracy that let a superbug claim 90 lives, http://www.dailymail.co.uk/health/article-487375/Cover-ups-lies-cynical-conspiracy-let-superbug-claim-90-lives.html, accessed 24 April 2010.

Clothier Inquiry (1994) *Independent Inquiry Relating to Deaths and Injuries on the Children's Ward at Grantham and Kesteven General Hospital*. London: HMSO.

Cochrane Collaboration (2011) *History*, http://www.cochrane.org/about-us/history, accessed 18 April 2011.

Cohen, S. (2002) *Folk Devils and Moral Panics: The Creation of the Mods and Rockers*. 3rd edition. London and New York: Routledge.

Community Care (Delayed Discharge Etc.) Act (2003)Chapter 5. http://www.opsi.gov.uk/acts/acts2003/en/ukpgaen_20030005_en_1.accesssed 22 June 2010.

Cooper, L., Coote, A., Davies, A. and Jackson, C. (1995) *Voices Off? Tackling the Democratic Deficit in Health*. London: Institute for Public Policy Research.

Couldry, N. (2000) *The Place of Media Power: Pilgrims and Witnesses of the Media Age*. London and New York: Routledge.

Coulter, A. (2002) After Bristol: putting patients at the centre. *BMJ*. 324: 648–51.

Coulter, A. (2005) What do patients and the public want from primary care? *BMJ*. 331: 1199–201.

Court of Appeal, Civil Division (1980) Whitehouse *v.* Jordan and another – [1980] 1 All ER 650.

Crinson, I. (2004) The politics of regulation within the 'modernized' NHS: the case of Beta interferon and the 'cost-effective' treatment of multiple sclerosis. *Critical Social Policy*. 24 (1): 30–49.

Crossman, R. H. S. (1977) *The Diaries of a Cabinet Minister*, Vol III. London: Hamish Hamilton and Jonathan Cape.

Croydon Area Health Authority (1976) *Report of the Committee of Inquiry Warlingham Park Hospital*. London: Croydon Area Health Authority.

Curtis, P. (2010) Budget 2010: public-sector cuts a 'declaration of war', say unions, *Guardian*, 22 June 2010, http://www.guardian.co.uk/uk/2010/jun/22/budget-public-sector-cuts-unions, accessed 19 April 2010.

Darzi, Sir Ara (2007) *A Framework for Action: Healthcare for London*, http://www.londonhp.nhs.uk/wp-content/uploads/2011/03/A-Framework-for-Action, accessed 29 June 2011.

Darzi, Professor the Lord of Denham (2008a) *High Quality Care for All: NHS Next Stage Review: Final Report*. Cm 7432. London: TSO, http://www.dh.gov.uk/en/Publicationsandstatistics/Publications/Publications PolicyAndGuidance/DH_085825, accessed 4 December 2008

Darzi, Professor the Lord of Denham (2008b) *Our NHS, Our Future*, http://www.networks.nhs.uk/news.php?nid=1802, accessed 18 July 2008.

Dearlove, J. and Saunders, P. (2000) *Introduction to British Politics*. 3rd edition. Cambridge and Oxford: Polity Press and Blackwell Publishers.

Defoe, D. (1722) *A journal of the plague year: being observations . . . of . . . occurences, . . . in London . . . in 1665 . . . by a citizen who continued all the while in London . . .* London: Printed for E. Nutt; J. Roberts; A. Dodd and J. Graves.

Department for Children, Schools and Families (2008a) Children's Trusts, statutory guidance on inter-agency cooperation to improve the well-being of children, young people and their families, http://www.everychild-matters.gov.uk/_files/48459BE8717A3D2E3C71501D44FA60BF.pdf, accessed 4 December 2008.

Department for the Environment Food and Rural Affairs (n.d.) Evidence based policy making, http://www.defra.gov.uk/science/how/evidence.htm, accessed 25 November 2008.

Department of Health (1989) *Working for Patients*. Cm 555. London: HMSO.

Department of Health (1991a) *The Health of the Nation. A Consultative Document for Health in England*. London: HMSO.

Department of Health (1991b) *The Patient's Charter*. London: HMSO.

Department of Health (1992) *The Health of the Nation. A Strategy for Health in England*. Cm 1986. London: HMSO.

Department of Health (1994) *Guidance on the Discharge of Mentally Disordered People and their Ccontinuing Care in the Community*. Health Service Guidelines, NHS Executive HSG(94)27, http://www.dh.gov.uk/prod_consum_dh/groups/dh_digitalassets/@dh/@en/documents/digital asset/dh_4120218.pdf, accessed 13 May 2010.

Department of Health (1997) *The New NHS: Modern, Dependable*. Cm 3807. London: HMSO.

Department of Health (1998a) *The Health of the Nation – A Policy Assessed*. London: TSO.

Department of Health (1998b) *A First Class Service – Quality in the New NHS*. [internet site]. Available: http://www.dh.gov.uk/assetRoot/04/04/49/41/04044941.pdf, accessed 11 November 2005.

Department of Health (1999a) *Saving Lives: Our Healthier Nation*. Cm 4386. London: TSO.

Department of Health (1999b) Report of the Expert Committee, Review of the 1983 Mental Health Act, http://www.dh.gov.uk/asset Root/04/02/12/00/04021200.pdf, accessed 15 November 2004.

Department of Health (1999c) *Clinical Governance: Quality in the New NHS*. London: Health Service Circular (1999/065).

Department of Health (2000a) *The NHS Plan: A Plan for Investment, a Plan for Reform*, http://www.dh.gov.uk/assetRoot/04/05/57/83/04055783.pdf, accessed 11 November 2005.

Department of Health (2000b) *An Organization with a Memory: Report of an Expert Group on Learning from Adverse Events in the NHS Chaired by the Chief Medical Officer*. London: TSO.

Department of Health (2000c) Reforming The Mental Health Act Part I. The New Legal Framework, http://www.archive.official-documents. co.uk/document/cm50/5016-i/5016i-02.htm, accessed 15 November 2004.

Department of Health (2001a) *Building a Safer NHS for Patients: Implementing an Organization with a Memory*. London: Department of Health.

Department of Health (2001b) *A Commitment to Quality, a Quest for Excellence. A Statement on behalf of the Government, the Medical Profession and the NHS*, http://www.dh.gov.uk/prod_consum_dh/groups/dh_ digitalassets/@dh/@en/documents/digitalasset/dh_4065056.pdf, accessed 29 November 2005

Department of Health (2002) *Shifting the Balance of Power – The Next Steps*. London: HMSO.

Department of Health (2003) *Building on the Best: Choice, Responsiveness and Equity in the NHS*. London: TSO.

Department of Health (2004a) *Improving Mental Health Law: Towards a New Mental Health Act. Summary*, http://www.dh.gov.uk/asset Root/04/08/89/18/04088918.pdf, accessed 15 November 2004.

Department of Health (2004b) *The NHS Improvement Plan: Putting People at the Heart of Public Services*. London: TSO.

Department of Health (2005a) *Independent Investigation of Adverse Events in Mental Health Services*. London: Department of Health, http://www.dh. gov.uk/prod_consum_dh/groups/dh_digitalassets/@dh/@en/documents/ digitalasset/dh_4113574.pdf, accessed 13 May 2010.

Department of Health (2005b) *Creating a Patient-Led NHS – Delivering the NHS Improvement Plan*, http://www.dh.gov.uk/en/Publicationsandstatistics/ Publications/PublicationsPolicyAndGuidance/DH_4106506, accessed 15 July 2006.

Department of Health (2006a) *Choice Matters: Increasing Choice Improves Patients' Experiences*. London: COI.

Department of Health (2006b) *Our Health, Our Care, Our Say*. London: Department of Health.

Department of Health (2007) Consultation, http://www.dh.gov.uk/
Consultations/fs/en, accessed 29 January 2007.

Department of Health (2008a) Ministers, http://www.dh.gov.uk/en/
Aboutus/MinistersandDepartmentLeaders/Ministers/index.htm, accessed
5 December 2008

Department of Health (2008b) Department leaders, http://www.dh.gov.
uk/en/Aboutus/MinistersandDepartmentLeaders/Departmentdirectors/
index.htm, accessed 9 December 2008

Department of Health (2010a) Anne Milton MP, http://www.dh.gov.uk/en/
Aboutus/MinistersandDepartmentLeaders/Ministers/Ministersbiography/
DH_116280, accessed 14 April 2011.

Department of Health (2010b) Ministerial responsibilities, http://www.
dh.gov.uk/en/Aboutus/MinistersandDepartmentLeaders/Ministers/
DH_116074, accessed 14 April 2011.

Department of Health (2010c) Andrew Lansley CBE MP http://www.
dh.gov.uk/en/Aboutus/MinistersandDepartmentLeaders/Ministers/
Ministersbiography/DH_115994, accessed 14 April 2011.

Department of Health (2010d) The role of national clinical directors,
http://www.dh.gov.uk/en/Aboutus/MinistersandDepartmentLeaders/
DH_4105389, accessed 15 April 2011.

Department of Health (2010e) DH Business Plan 2011–2015: consultation
on the Transparency Framework, http://www.dh.gov.uk/en/Consultations/
Closedconsultations/DH_122220, accessed 22 April 2011.

Department of Health (2011a) How DH works, http://www.dh.gov.uk/en/
Aboutus/HowDHworks/index.htm, accessed 15 April 2011.

Department of Health (2011b) Chief Medical Officer, http://www.dh.gov.
uk/en/Aboutus/MinistersandDepartmentLeaders/ChiefMedicalOfficer/
index.htm, accessed 15 April 2011.

Department of Health (2011c) Departmental Board, http://www.dh.gov.uk/
en/Aboutus/HowDHworks/BoardsandCommittees/DepartmentalBoard/
index.htm., accessed 18 April 2011

Department of Health (2011d) Ministers and Department leaders,
http://www.dh.gov.uk/en/Aboutus/MinistersandDepartmentLeaders/index.htm,
accessed 15 April 2011.

Department of Health and Social Security (1971) *Better Services for the
Mentally Handicapped.* Cmnd 4683. London: HMSO.

Department of Health and Social Security (1975) *Better Services for the
Mentally Ill.* Cmnd 6233. London: HMSO.

Department of Health and Social Security (1976a) *Priorities for Health and
Personal Social Services in England: A Consultative Document.* London:
HMSO

Department of Health and Social Security (1976b) *Sharing Resources
for Health in England: Report of the Resource Allocation Working Parties.*
London: Department of Health and Social Security.

Department of Health and Social Security and the Welsh Office (1978) *A*

Happier Old Age: A Discussion Document on Elderly People in Our Society. London: HMSO.

Department of Health and Social Security (1980) *Report of the Review of Rampton Hospital.* Cmnd 8073. London: HMSO.

Department of Health and Social Security (1981) *Drinking Sensibly: A Discussion Document Prepared by the Health Departments of Great Britain and Northern Ireland.* London: Department of Health and Social Security.

Department of Health and Social Security (1982) *Child Abuse: A Study of Inquiry Reports.* London: HMSO.

Dolbeare K. M. and Cummings, M. S. (2004) *American Political Thought.* 5th edition. Washington: CQ Press.

Donaldson, Sir Liam (2008) About the Chief Medical Officer (CMO), http://www.dh.gov.uk/en/Aboutus/MinistersandDepartmentLeaders/ ChiefMedicalOfficer/AboutTheChiefMedicalOfficerCMO/index.htm, accessed 8 December 2008.

Donaldson, Sir Liam (2010) Passive drinking: the collateral damage from alcohol. In *Annual Report of the Chief Medical officer: On the State of Public Health 2008.* London: Department of Health, http:/www.dh.gov.uk/prod_ consum_dh/groups/dh_digitalassets/documents/digitalassets/dh_096229. pdf, accessed 27 May 2010.

Douglas, M. (1990) Risk as a forensic resource. *Dædalus. Journal of the American Academy of Arts and Sciences.* 119 (4): 1–16.

Douglas, M. (1992) *Risk and Blame: Essays in Cultural Theory.* London: Routledge.

Drewry, G. (1996) Judicial inquiries and public reassurance. *Public Law.* 368–83.

Dror, Y. (1964) 'Muddling through' — 'science' or inertia? *Public Administration Review,* 24: 135–57.

Dror, Y. (1987) Conclusions. In *Advising The Rulers,* ed. W. Plowden. Oxford: Basil Blackwell, pp. 185–215.

Dye, T. R. (1976) *Policy Analysis.* Alabama: University of Alabama Press.

Dyer, C. (2005) Shipman inquiry finds GMC has 'fundamental flaws'. *BMJ.* 330 (7481): 10.

Eagleton, T. (1994) *Ideology: An Introduction.* London: Verso.

Eatwell, R. (1993) Introduction: what are political ideologies? In *Contemporary Political Ideologies,* ed. R. Eatwell and A. Wright. London: Continuum, pp. 1–22.

Eckstein, H. (1960) *Pressure Group Politics: The Case of the British Medical Association.* London: Allen & Unwin.

Eldridge, J. (1993) News, truth and power. In *Getting the Message: News, Truth and Power,* ed. J. Eldridge. London and New York: Routledge.

Encyclopædia Britannica (2010) Romanticism, http://www.britannica.com/ EBchecked/topic/508675/Romanticism, accessed 10 June 2010.

Evans-Pritchard, E. E. (1976) *Witchcraft, Oracles and Magic among the Azande.* Oxford: Clarendon Press.

Expert Advisory Group on Cancer (2005) *A Report by the Expert Advisory Group on Cancer to the Chief Medical Officers of England and Wales: A Policy Framework for Commissioning Cancer services, Guidance for Purchasers and Providers of Cancer Services*, April 2005, http://www.dh.gov.uk/asset-Root/04/06/38/20/04063820.pdf, accessed 15 January 2007.

Fenn, P., Diacon, S., Gray, A., Hodges, R. and Rickman, N. (2000) Current cost of medical negligence in NHS hospitals, analysis of claims database. *BMJ*. 320: 1567–71.

Fenn, P., Hermans, D. and Dingwall, R. (1994) Estimating the cost of compensating victims of medical negligence. *BMJ*. 309: 389–91.

Ferlie, E., Freeman, G., McDonnell, J., Petsoulas, C. and Rundle-Smith, S. (2006) Introducing choice in the public services: some supply-side issues. *Public Money and Management*. 26 (1): 63–72.

Ferriman, A. (2000) The stigma of schizophrenia. *BMJ*. 320: 522.

Flynn, R. (2002) Clinical governance and governmentality. *Health, Risk and Society*. 4 (2): 155–70.

Foucault, M. (1984) Space, knowledge and power. In *The Foucault Reader*, ed. P. Rabinow. New York: Pantheon, pp. 239–56.

Foucault, M. (1988) On problematization, *History of the Present*. 4: 16–17.

Fowler, N. (1991) *Ministers Decide: A Personal Memoir of the Thatcher Years*. London: Chapmans.

Frank, A. (2000) *Notes on Habermas: Lifeworld and System*, http://www.ucalgary.ca/~frank/habermas.html, accessed 18 November 2006.

Freedman, D. (2002) Clinical governance – bridging management and clinical approaches to quality in the UK. *Clinica Chimica Acta*. 319: 133–41.

Fukuyama, F. (1992) *The End of History and the Last Man*. New York: Free Press.

Furedi, F. (2002) *Culture of Fear: Risk Taking and the Morality of Low Expectation*. London: Cassell.

Furedi, F. (2004) *Therapy Culture: Cultivating Vulnerability in an Uncertain Age*. London: Routledge.

Furedi, F. (2005) *Politics of Fear: Beyond Left and Right*. London: Continuum.

Gann, R. (1995) The limits of textbook ideology. *Politics*. 15 (2): 127–33.

Giddens, A. (1990) *The Consequences of Modernity*. Cambridge: Polity.

Giddens, A. (1994) *Beyond Left and Right: The Future of Radical Politics*. Stanford: Stanford University Press.

Gilleard, C. and Higgs, P. (2000) *Cultures of Ageing: Self, Citizen and the Body*. Harlow: Prentice Hall.

Glendinning, L. and Tran, M. (2008) *Balls Orders Urgent Inquiry into Baby P Case*, http://www.guardian.co.uk/society/2008/nov/12/childprotection-climbie, accessed 10 March 2010.

Gordon, A. (1993) Twenty-two theses on social constructionism: a feminist response to Ibarra and Kitsuse's 'Proposal for the study of social problems'. In *Reconsidering Social Constructionism: Debates in Social Problems Theory*, ed. J. Holstein and G. Miller. New York: Aldine de Gruyter, pp. 301–26.

Gregory, R. (1993) Political rationality or incrementalism. In *The Policy Process: A Reader*, ed. M. Hill. New York: Harvester/Wheatsheaf.

Gustafsson, G. (1983) Symbolic and pseudo policies as responses to diffusion of power. *Policy Sciences*. 15: 269–87.

Habermas, J. (1984) *Theory of Communicative Action*, Vol. I: *Reason and the Rationalization of Society*. Cambridge: Polity.

Habermas, J. (1987) *Theory of Communicative Action*, Vol. II: *Lifeworld and System: A Critique of Functionalist Reason*. Cambridge: Polity.

Habermas, J. (1989) *The Structural Transformation of the Public Sphere: An Inquiry into a Category of Bourgeois Society*. Cambridge, Mass.: MIT Press.

Hailsham, Lord (1976) Elective dictatorship, *The Listener*, 496–500, 21 October 1976.

Hale, M. (1713) *The History of the Common Law of England*, reprinted http://www.efm.bris.ac.uk/het/hale/common, accessed 6 October 2008.

Hall, P., Land, H., Parker, R. and Webb, A. (1975) *Change, Choice and Conflict in Social Policy*. London: Heinemann, pp.124–55.

Hall, S. (1991) The rediscovery of 'ideology': return of the repressed in media studies. In *Mass Media and Society*, ed. J. Curran, M. Gurevitch and J. Woollacott. London: Edward Arnold.

Ham, C. (2004) *Health Policy in Britain: The Politics and Organization of the National Health Service*. 5th edition. Basingstoke: Palgrave Macmillan.

Ham, C. and Hill, M. (1993) *The Policy Process in the Modern Capitalist State*. 2nd edition. New York: Harvester Wheatsheaf.

Harrison, S. and Smith, C. (2004) Trust and moral motivation: redundant resources in health and social care. *Policy and Politics*. 32 (3): 371–86.

Haywood, S. and Alaszewski, A. (1980) *Crisis in the Health Service: The Politics of Management*. London: Croom Helm.

Heald, D. (1983) *Public Expenditure: Its Defence and Reform*. Oxford: Martin Robertson.

Heclo, H. and Wildavsky, A. (1974) *The Private Government of Public Money: Community and Policy inside British Politics*. London: Macmillan.

Heclo, H. and Wildavsky, A. (1981) *The Private Government of Public Money: Community and Policy inside British Politics*. 2nd edition. London: Macmillan.

Hedgecoe, A. (2004) *The Politics of Personalised Medicine: Pharmacogenetics in the Clinic*. Cambridge: Cambridge University Press.

Heffernan, R. (2000) *New Labour and Thatcherism*. Basingstoke: Macmillan.

Hegemann, W. (1929) *Frederick the Great*. London: Constable.

Hennessy, P. (1990) *Whitehall*. London: Fontana Press.

Hennock, E. P. (1998) Vaccination policy against smallpox, 1835–1914: a comparison of England with Prussia and Imperial Germany. *Social History of Medicine*. 11: 49–71.

Her Majesty's Government (1966) *Report of the Royal Commission on Tribunals of Inquiry*. Cmnd 3121. London: HMSO.

Her Majesty's Government (1999) *Modernising Government*. Cm 4310. London: TSO, http://www.archive.official-documents.co.uk/document/cm43/4310/4310.htm, accessed 25 September 2007.

Her Majesty's Treasury (n.d.) *Spending Review: Public Expenditure Planning and Control in the UK*, http://www.hm-treasury.gov.uk/spend_plancontrol. htm, accessed 28 July 2009 and 17 August 2009.

Her Majesty's Treasury (1998) Current and capital spending: a vital distinction in the fiscal framework, Press Release, http://www.hm-treasury.gov. uk/press_93_98.htm, accessed 12 August 2009.

Her Majesty's Treasury (2000a) *Department of Health, 2000 Spending Review: Public Services Agreement White Paper*, http://www.hm-treasury. gov.uk/pss_psa_doh.htm, accessed 13 August 2009.

Her Majesty's Treasury (2005) *The Golden Rule*, http://www.hm-treasury. gov.uk/foi_goldenrule_010205.htm, accessed 5 August 2009.

Her Majesty's Treasury (2006) *Long-term Opportunities and Challenges for the UK: Analysis for the 2007 Comprehensive Spending Review*, http://www. hm-treasury.gov.uk/d/csr_longterm271106.pdf, accessed 4 August 2009.

Her Majesty's Treasury (2007) *Meeting the Aspirations of the British People, Pre-Budget Report and Comprehensive Spending Review*. Cm 7227. London: TSO, http://www.hm-treasury.gov.uk/d/pbr_csr07_completereport_1546. pdf, accessed 17 August 2009.

Her Majesty's Treasury (2009) Spending reviews, http://www.hm-treasury. gov.uk/spend_index.htm, accessed 12 August 2009.

Her Majesty's Treasury (2010) *Spending Review 2010*. Cm 7942. London: TSO,   http://cdn.hm-treasury.gov.uk/sr2010_completereport.pdf, accessed 19 April 2011.

Herxheimer, A. (2003) Relationships between the pharmaceutical industry and patients' organizations. *BMJ*. 326: 1208–10.

Heyman, B., Shaw, M.. Alaszewski, A. and Titterton, M. (2009) *Risk, Safety and Clinical Practice: Health Care through the Lens of Risk*. Oxford: Oxford University Press.

Heywood, A. (2007) *Political Ideologies: An Introduction*. London: Palgrave.

Hickson, K. (2005) *The IMF Crisis of 1976 and British Politics: Keynesian Social Democracy, Monetarism and Economic Liberalism: the 1970s Struggle in British Politics*. London: Tauris Academic Studies.

Hill, R. (2008) *God's Architect: Pugin and the Building of Romantic Britain*. London: Penguin Books.

Ho, L. (2006) Constitutional democracy, representation, and governance. Paper presented at 'Constitutional Democracy, Representation, and Governance', Chinese University of Hong Kong, Hong Kong. 14–17 December.

Holstein, J. and G. Miller. (1993) Reconstituting the constructionist program. In *Reconsidering Social Constructionism: Debates in Social Problems Theory*, ed. J. Holstein and G. Miller. New York: Aldine de Gruyter, pp. 253–80.

Holt, J.C. (1992) *The Magna Carta,*. 2nd edition. Cambridge: Cambridge University Press.

Hood, C. (2005) Discussant of: M. Calnan and R. Rowe – *Trust Relations in the New NHS: Theoretical and Methodological Challenges*. Paper presented at 'Taking Stock of Trust'. LSE. 12 December 2005.

Horlick-Jones, T. (2005) On 'risk work': professional discourse, account-ability and everyday action. *Health, Risk and Society*. 7 (3): 293–307.

House of Commons (2001) *Report. The Royal Liverpool Children's Inquiry*. London: HMSO, http://www.rlcinquiry.org.uk/download/index.htm, accessed 14 May 2010.

House of Commons, Science and Technology Committee (2006) *Scientific Advice, Risk and Evidence Based Policy Making*, Seventh Report of Session 2005–6, Vol. I, Ordered by The House of Commons to be printed 26 October 2006, http://www.publications.parliament.uk/pa/cm200506/cmselect/cmsctech/900/900-i.pdf, accessed 13 April 2010.

House of Commons Health Committee (2005) The influence of the phar-maceutical industry, http://www.parliament.the-stationery-office.co.uk/pa/cm200405/cmselect/cmhealth/42/42.pdf, accessed 30 March 2010.

Hughes, E., Kitzinger, J. and Murdock, G. (2004) The media and risk. In *Risk in Social Science*, ed. P. Taylor-Gooby and J. O. Zinn. Oxford: Oxford University Press, pp. 250–70.

Iannucci, A. (2010) A new politics? Not until we blow away the rhetorical smokescreens. *The Independent*, 5 June 2010.

Illich, I. (1976) *Limits to Medicine*. London: Marion Boyars.

Jayasuriya, K. (2001) September 11 and the new 'anti-politics' of 'security'. *Australian Review of Public Affairs Digest*, 8 December 2001.

Jenkins, W. I (1978) *Policy Analysis: A Political and Organizational Perspective*. London: Martin Robertson.

Jermier, J (1988). Introduction: critical perspective on organizational control. *Administrative Science Quarterly*. 43: 235–56.

Jessop, B. (2006) *From Thatcherism to New Labour: Neo-Liberalism, Workfarism, and Labour Market Regulation*. Lancaster: Department of Sociology, Lancaster University, http://www.comp.lancs.ac.uk/sociology/soc131rj.pdf, accessed 12 December 2009.

Jesudason, J. (1999) The resilience of one-party dominance in Malaysia and Singapore. In *The Awkward Embrace: One-Party Domination and Democracy*, ed. H. Giliomee and C. Simkins. Australia: Harwood Academic Publishers, pp. 127–71.

Jonas, H. (1984) *The Imperative of Responsibility. In Search of an Ethics for the Technological Age*. Chicago: University of Chicago Press.

Jones, I. (2001) Health care decision making and the politics of health. In *Habermas, Critical Theory and Health*, ed. G. Scambler. London: Routledge, pp. 68–85.

Jones, K. (1972) *A History of the Mental Health Services*. London and Boston: Routledge and Kegan Paul.

Jones, K. (1993) *Asylums and After: A Revised History of the Mental Health Services*. London: Athlone Press.

Jones, K. and Fowles, A. J. (1984) *Ideas on Institutions: Analysing the Literature on Long-term Care and Custody*. London: Routledge and Kegan Paul.

Katwala, S., Whitford, B. and Ottery, C. (2003) Politics and the media: is it time for change? *Observer*, Sunday 27 July 2003, http://www.guardian.co.uk/politics/2003/jul/27/media.davidkelly, accessed 8 April 2010.

Kavanagh, D., Richards, D., Geddes, A. and Smith, M. (2006) *British Politics*. Oxford: Oxford University Press.

Kemshall, H. (2002) *Risk, Social Policy and Welfare*. Buckingham: Open University Press.

Kennedy, H. (2004) *Just Law: The Changing Face of Justice – and Why it Matters to us All*. London: Secker & Warburg.

Kewell, B. J. (2006) Language games and tragedy: the Bristol Royal Infirmary disaster revisited. *Health, Risk and Society*. 8: 359–77.

Keynes, J. M. (1973) *The General Theory of Employment, Interest and Money, the Collected Writings*, Vol. VII. London: Macmillan, http://homepage.newschool.edu/het//texts/keynes/chap24.htm, accessed 4 August 2009.

Kingdom, J. (1991) *Government and Politics in Britain: An Introduction*. Cambridge: Polity Press.

Kingdom, J. (1999) *Government and Politics in Britain: An Introduction*. 2nd edition. Cambridge: Polity.

Kingdon, J. (1995) *Agendas, Alternatives and Public Policies*. 2nd edition. Harlow: Longman.

Kitzinger, J. (1999) Researching risk and the media. *Health, Risk and Society*. 1: 55–69.

Kitzinger, J. (2004) *Framing Abuse: Media Influence and Public Understanding of Sexual Violence against Children*. London and Ann Arbor, Mich.: Pluto Press.

Kitzinger, J (2006) The media and risk. In *Risk in the Social Sciences*, ed. P. Taylor-Gooby and J. O. Zinn. Oxford: Oxford University Press, pp. 160–79.

Klaassen, B., Buckley, J. R. and Esmail, A. (1996) Does the Dangerous Dogs Act protect against animal attacks: a prospective study of mammalian bites in the Accident and Emergency Department. *Injury*. 27 (2): 89–91.

Klein, R. (1998) Why Britain is reorganizing its national health service – yet again. *Health Affairs*. 17 (4): 111–25.

Klein, R. (2001) *The New Politics of the National Health Service*. 4th edition. Harlow: Prentice Hall.

Kumlin, S. and Rothstein, B. (2005) Making and breaking social capital: the impact of welfare state institutions. *Comparative Political Studies*. 38 (4): 339–65.

Lam, A. (2000) Tacit knowledge, organizational learning and societal institutions – an integrated framework. *Organizational Studies*. 21: 487–513.

Laming, Lord (2003) *Report of an Inquiry by Lord Laming. The Victoria Climbié Inquiry*. Cm 5730. London: HMSO.

TheLancet.com (n.d.) About the Lancet medical journal, http://www.the-lancet.com/lancet-about, accessed 5 March 2010.

Laurance, J. (2003) *Pure Madness: How fear drives the mental health system*. London: Routledge.

Law, A. (2008) The elixir of social trust: social capital and cultures of challenge in health movements. In *Researching Trust and Health*, ed. J. Brownlie, A. Greene and A. Howson. London: Routledge, pp.175–93.

Lawson, N. (1993) *The View from No. 11: Memoirs of a Tory Radical*. London: Corgi.

Le Grand, J. (2007) *The Other Invisible Hand: Delivering Public Services through Choice and Competition*. Princeton: Princeton University Press.

Lewis, T. (2006) Zero-based budgeting. *eGov Monitor*, http://www.egov-monitor.com/node/4886/print, accessed 29 July 2009.

Liberal Democrats (2010) Conservative Liberal Democrat coalition agreements, 12 May 2010, http://www.libdems.org.uk/latest_news_detail.aspx?title=Conservative_Liberal_Democrat_coalition_agreements&pPK=2697bcdc-7483-47a7-a517-7778979458ff, accessed 19 April 2011.

Lindblom, C. (1959) The science of 'muddling through'. *Public Administration Review*. 19: 79–88.

Lindblom, C. (1979) Still muddling, not yet through. *Public Administration Review*. 39: 517–26.

Lodge, M. and Hood, C. (2002) Pavlovian policy responses to media feeding frenzies? Dangerous dogs regulation in comparative perspective. *Journal of Contingencies and Crisis Management*. 10 (1): 1–13.

Lowe, R. (1997) Milestone or millstone? The 1959–1961 Plowden Committee and its impact on British welfare policy. *Historical Journal*. 40: 463–91.

McKeown, T. (1979) *The Role of Medicine: Dream, Mirage, Nemesis?* Princeton: Princeton University Press.

Mairal, G. (2011) A narrative structure of risk in the media. *Health, Risk and Society*. 13: 65–79.

Marcuse, H. (1989) From ontology to technology: fundamental tendencies of industrial society. In *Critical Theory and Society: A Reader*, ed. S. Bronner and D. Kellner. London: Routledge, pp. 119–29.

Martin, J. P. with Evans, D. (1984) *Hospitals in Trouble*. Oxford: Basil Blackwell.

Marx, K. and Engels, F. (1977) *The German Ideology: Part One*. London: Lawrence and Wishart.

Maynard, A. (2003) An economic approach to clinical governance. In *Clinical Governance and Best Value: Meeting the Modernization Agenda*, ed.

S. Pickering and J. Thompson. Edinburgh: Churchill Livingstone, pp. 17–32.

Means, R. and Smith, R. (1985) *The Development of Welfare Services for Elderly People*. London: Croom Helm.

Mechanic, D. (1995) Dilemmas in rationing health care services: the case for implicit rationing. *BMJ*. 310: 1655–9.

Mental Health Act (1995) Mental Health (Patients in the Community) Act Chapter 52. London: HMSO.

Mental Health Act (2003) Mental Health Act. Chapter 20, http://www. cqc.org.uk/_db/_documents/Mental_Health_Act_1983_201005272747. pdf, accessed 31 May 2010.

Mental Health Act (2007) Mental Health Act. Chapter 12, http://www.opsi. gov.uk/acts/acts2007/ukpga_20070012_en_1, accessed 31 May 2010.

Mill, J. S. (1993) *On Liberty and Utilitarianism*. New York: Bantam.

Miller, D. and Williams, K. (1993) Negotiating HIV/AIDS information: agendas, media strategies and news. In *Getting the Message: News, Truth and Power*, ed. J. Eldridge. London and New York: Routledge, pp. 126–42.

Mind (2004) Submission to the Joint Committee on the Draft Mental Health Bill: summary, http://www.mind.org.uk/NR/rdonlyres/1BC535C1-3CB3-4BBF-81F2-09543AA3E668/0/SummaryofMindsubmissionto JointCommittee.pdf, accessed 15 November 2004.

Moncrieff, J. (2003) Is psychiatry for sale?: an examination of the influence of the pharmaceutical industry on academic and practical psychiatry. Maudesley Discussion Paper # 13, http://www.iop.kcl.ac.uk/ departments/?locator=528, accessed 30 March 2010.

Moran, M. (2003) *The British Regulatory State: High Modernism and Hyper-Innovation*. Oxford: Oxford University Press.

MORI (2004) *In Search of Lost Trust*. London: MORI.

Munro, N (2005) What can policy makers learn from homicide inquiries? http://www.lse.ac.uk/collections/CARR/pdf/05StudentConf/Munro.pdf, accessed 13 April 2010.

National Council for Civil Liberties (1951) *50,000 Outside the Law: Report of the Treatment of Those Certified as Mental Defectives*. London: NCCL.

National Health Executive (2011) Ministers promise change to NHS reforms. 6 April 2011, http://www.nationalhealthexecutive.com/Ministers-promise-change-to-NHS-reforms.htm, accessed 14 April 2011.

National Institute for Health Research (n.d.) Patient and Public Involvement (PPI), http://www.ccf.nihr.ac.uk/PPI/Pages/default.aspx, accessed 22 April 2011.

National Health Service (1968) *Findings and Recommendations following Enquiries into Allegations concerning the Care of Elderly Patients in Certain Hospitals*. Cmnd 3689. London: HMSO.

National Health Service (1969) *Report of the Committee of Inquiry into Allegations of Ill-Treatment of Patients and Other Irregularities at Ely Hospital, Cardiff*. Cmnd 3975. London: HMSO.

National Health Service (1971) *Report of the Farleigh Hospital Committee of Inquiry*. Cmnd 3975. London: HMSO.
National Health Service (1972a) *Report of the Committee Appointed to Inquire into the Circumstances, including the Production, which Led to the Use of Contaminated Infusion Fluids in the Devonport Section of Plymouth General Hospital*. Cmnd 5035. London: HMSO.
National Health Service (1972b) *Report of the Committee of Inquiry into Whittingham Hospital*. Cmnd 4861. London: HMSO.
National Health Service (1978) *Report of the Committee of Inquiry into Normansfield Hospital*. Cmnd 7357. London: HMSO.
National Health Service (1992) *Report of the Committee of Inquiry into Complaints about Ashworth Hospital*. Cmnd 2028. London: HMSO.
National Health Service (1999) *Report of the Committee of Inquiry into the Personality Disorder Unit, Ashworth Special Hospital*, Vol. I. Cm 4194-ii. London: TSO.
National Health Service (2010) National service frameworks and strategies, http://www.nhs.uk/NHSEngland/NSF/Pages/Nationalserviceframeworks. aspx, accessed 27 April 2010.
National Health Service Executive (1999) Clinical governance in the new NHS, Health Service Circular, HSC 2000/065. Leeds: Department of Health.
National Health Service London (2010a) Independent Inquiries, http:// www.london.nhs.uk/publications/independent-publications/independent-inquiries, accessed 16 May 2010.
National Health Service London (2010b) Health and Social Care Advisory Service Report of the independent investigation into the care and treatment of Mr BM: a report for NHS London, http://www.london.nhs. uk/webfiles/Corporate/Mental%20Health%20reports/Legacy/BMReport. pdf, accessed 27 April 2010 and 17 June 2010.
National Health Service Management Executive (1992) *Local Voices. The Views of Local People in Purchasing for Health*. London: Department of Health.
National Health Service Wales / GIG Cymru (n.d.) NHS prescription charges, Health of Wales, Information Services, http://www.wales.nhs.uk/ page.cfm?pid=9586, accessed 26 November 2008.
Navarro, V. (1978) *Class Struggle, The State and Medicine: An Historical and Contemporary Analysis of the Medical Sector in Great Britain*. London: Martin Robertson.
Negrine, R. (1994) *Politics and the Mass Media in Britain*. 2nd edition. London and New York: Routledge.
Newman, A. and Vidler, E. (2006) Discriminating customers, responsible patients, empowered users: consumerism and the modernization of health care. *Journal of Social Policy*. 35 (2): 193–209.
NICE (2008a) About NICE, http://www.nice.org.uk/aboutnice/about_nice. jsp, accessed 9 December 2008.
NICE (2008b) Social value judgements: principles for the development

of NICE guidance. 2nd edition, http://www.nice.org.uk/media/C18/30/ SVJ2PUBLICATION2008.pdf, accessed 9 December 2008.

Northcote, S. H. and Trevelyan, C. E. (1854) Report on the Organisation of the Permanent Civil Service presented to both Houses of parliament by Command of her Majesty, Her Majesty's Stationery Office, London, http://www.civilservant.org.uk/northcotetrevelyan.pdf, accessed 28 June 2011.

Northern Ireland Executive (2008) 02 April 2008 – Health minister announces freeze on prescription charges, http://www.northernireland. gov.uk/news-dhssps-020408-health-minister-announces, accessed 26 November 2008.

Nottinghamshire Healthcare National Health Service (n.d.) Rampton Hospital, http://nottinghamshirehealthcare.nhs.uk/our-services/forensic-services/rampton- hospital, accessed 11 May 2010.

Number 10 (2010) PM visits Cumbria, http://www.number10.gov.uk/news/ latest-news/2010/06/pm-visits-cumbria-51382, accessed 17 June 2010.

O'Grady, S. (2011) NHS Pledge distorts the Coalition's spending choices. *The Independent*, 18 April 2011.

Oliver, J. and Oakeshott, L. (2008) Secret papers reveal Tony Blair's F1 tobacco deal. *The Sunday Times*, 12 October 2008, http://www.timeson-line.co.uk/tol/news/politics/article4926737.ece, accessed 9 April 2010.

Osborne, D. and Gaebler, T. (1992) *Reinventing Government*. Reading, Mass.: Addison-Wesley.

Osborne, J. and Osborne, O. (2005) Regulating doctors: should we swallow Dame Janet's medicine? *BMJ*. 330: 546.

Osborne, S. P. and McLaughlin, K. (2000) The New Public Management in context. In *The New Public Management, Current Trends and Future Prospects*, ed. K. McLaughlin, S. P. Osborne and E. Ferlie. London: Routledge, pp. 7–14.

Osborne, T. (1997) Of health and statecraft. In *Foucault, Health and Medicine*, ed. A. Petersen and R. Bunton. London: Routledge, pp. 173–88.

The Oxford Dictionary of Economics (n.d.) Stop–go cycle, http://www.enotes. com/econ-encyclopedia/stop-go-cycle, accessed 5 August 2009.

Parkinson, J. (2009) Pledge watch: dangerous dogs. *BBC News* 4 December 2009, http://news.bbc.co.uk/?1/hi/uk_politics/8391175.stm, accessed 12 April 2010.

Paroske, M. (2005) The rhetoric of AIDS policy in South Africa. Ph.D thesis. Pittsburgh: University of Pittsburgh, http://etd.library.pitt.edu/ ETD/available/etd-04182006-133611/unrestricted/Paroskediss.pdf.

Parry, N. and Parry, J. (1976) *The Rise of the Medical Profession: A Study of Collective Social Mobility*. London: Croom Helm.

Parsons, T. (1949) *Structure of Social Action: A Study in Social Theory with Special Reference to a Group of Recent European Writers*. New York: Free Press of Glencoe.

Perrow, C. (1999) *Normal Accidents: Living with High-Risk Technologies.* Princeton: Princeton University Press.

Peterson, A. (1997) Risk, governance and the new public health. In *Foucault, Health and Medicine*, ed. A. Petersen and R. Bunton. London: Routledge, pp 189–206.

Philo, G. (1999) Media and mental illness. In *Message Received: Glasgow Media Group Research 1993–1998*, ed. G. Philo. Harlow: Longman.

Philo, G., McLaughlin, G. and Henderson, L. (1996) Media content. In *Media and Mental Distress*, ed. G. Philo. London: Longman, pp. 45–81.

Pickering, M. (2001) *Stereotyping – The Politics of Representation.* Basingstoke: Palgrave.

Pickering, S. and Thompson, J. (eds.) (2003) *Clinical Governance and Best Value: Meeting the Modernization Agenda.* Edinburgh: Churchill Livingstone.

Pidgeon, N., Kasperson, R.E. and Slovic, P. (eds.) (2003) *The Social Amplification of Risk.* Cambridge: Cambridge University Press.

Pieterman, R. (2005) The 'risk society' or a 'precautionary culture'. SSPSSR Lecture. University of Kent. 17 November 2005.

Pilgrim, D. (2007) New 'mental health' legislation for England and Wales: some aspects of consensus and conflict. *Journal of Social Policy.* 36: 79–95.

Pilgrim, D. (2008) Reading 'happiness': CBT and the Layard thesis. *European Journal of Psychotherapy & Counselling.* 10 (3): 247–60.

Plato (2003) *The Republic.* London: Penguin.

Pollard, J. (2011) Seen, seared and sealed: trauma and the visual presentation of September 11th. *Health, Risk and Society.* 13: 81–101.

Pontusson, J. (1997) Between neo-liberalism and the German model: Swedish capitalism in transition. In *Political Economy of Modern Capitalism*, ed. C. Crouch and W. Streeck. Thousand Oaks, Calif.: Sage, pp. 55–70.

Powell, M. (2000) New Labour and the third way in the British welfare state: a new and distinctive approach? *Critical Social Policy.* 20: 39–60.

Powell, T. and Gay, O. (2004) *Individual Ministerial Responsibility – Issues and Examples.* Research Paper, 04/31, Parliament and Constitution Centre, House of Commons, http://www.parliament.uk/commons/lib/research/rp2004/rp04-031.pdf, accessed 29 November 2008.

Power, M. (2003) Evaluating the audit explosion. *Law and Policy.* 25: 185–202.

Power, M. (2004) *The Risk Management of Everything: Rethinking the Politics of Uncertainty.* London: Demos.

Power, M. (2007) *Organized Uncertainty: Designing a World of Risk Management.* Oxford: Oxford University Press.

Price, K. (2010) Towards a history of medical negligence. *Lancet.* 375. 9710: 192–93. 16 January 2010, http://www.thelancet.com/journals/lancet/article/PIIS0140-6736(10)60081-5/fulltext, accessed 10 May 2010.

Public Interest Disclosure Act (1998) Chapter 23, http:/www.opsi.gov.uk/acts/acts1998/ukpga_19980023_en_1 accessed 29 April 2010.

Queens Bench Division (1957) Bolam *v.* Friern Hospital Management

Committee, http://oxcheps.new.ox.ac.uk/casebook/Resources/BOLAMV_ 1% 20DOC.pdf, accessed 17 June 2010.

Rees, R. (2001) *Poverty and Public Health, 1815–1948*. Oxford: Heinemann.

Reilly, J. (1999) 'Just another food scare?' Public understanding and the BSE crisis. In *Message Received: Glasgow Media Group Research 1993–1998*, ed. G. Philo. Harlow: Longman, pp. 128–46.

Rhodes, R. A. W. (1997) *Understanding Government: Policy Networks, Governance and Accountability*. Buckingham and New York: Open University Press.

Richards, D. and Smith, M. (2002) *Governance and Public Policy in the UK*. Oxford: Oxford University Press.

Riesch, H. and Spiegelhalter, D (2011) Careless pork costs lives: risk stories from science to press release to media. *Health, Risk and Society*. 13(1): 46–67.

Ritchie Inquiry (1994) *Report of the Inquiry into the Care and Treatment of Christopher Clunis*, Chairman J. H. Ritchie. London: HMSO.

Robb, B. (ed.) (1967) *Sans Everything*. Edinburgh: Thomas Nelson.

Rose, R. (1996) Steering the ship of state. In *The Whitehall Reader: The UK's Administrative Machine in Action*, ed. P. Barberis. Buckingham: Open University Press, pp. 103–10.

Rose, R., Mishler, W. and Haerpfer, C. (1998) *Democracy and Its Alternatives: Understanding Post-Communist Societies*. Baltimore: Johns Hopkins University Press.

Rothstein, H. (2006) The institutional origins of risk: a new agenda for risk research. *Health, Risk and Society*. 8 (3): 215–21.

Rousseau, J.-J. (2008) [1762] *The Social Contract*. New York: Cosimo.

Rowe, R. and Shepherd, M. (2002) Public participation in the New NHS: no closer to citizen control. *Social Policy and Administration*. 36 (3): 275–90.

Royal College of Physicians (2008) More details on our vision, purpose and objectives, http://www.rcplondon.ac.uk/About-the-college/Pages/mission-purpose-details.aspx, accessed 3 December 2008.

Royal Commission on the Law Relating to Mental Illness and Mental Deficiency (1957) *Report*. Cmnd 169. London: HMSO.

Royal Pharmaceutical Society of Great Britain (2008) *Frequently Asked Questions about Prescription Charges*, http://www.rpsgb.org.uk/pdfs/pre-scriptioncharges.pdf, accessed on 28 November 2008.

Sanders, D., Marsh, D. and Ward, H. (1993) The electoral impact of press coverage of the British economy, 1979–87. *British Journal of Political Studies*. 23: 175–210.

SANE (2008) About SANE, http://www.sane.org.uk/AboutSANE, accessed December 2008.

Saunders, P. (1984) Rethinking local politics. In *Local Socialism: The Way Forward*, ed. M. Boddy and C. Fudge. London: Macmillan, pp. 22–48.

Scally, G. and Donaldson, L. (1998) Clinical governance and the drive for quality improvement in the new NHS in England. *BMJ*. 317: 61–5.

Scambler, G. (2001) Introduction: unfolding themes of an incomplete project. In *Habermas, Critical Theory and Health*, ed. G. Scambler. London: Routledge, pp. 1–24.

Scambler, G. and Britten, N. (2001) System, lifeworld and doctor–patient interaction: issues of trust in a changing world. In *Habermas, Critical Theory and Health*, ed. G. Scambler. London: Routledge, pp. 45–64.

Schieder, F. (2000) *Frederick the Great*. London: Penguin.

Schutz, A. (1964) *Collected Papers*, Vol. II: *Studies in Social Theory*, ed. and tr. Arvid Brodersen. The Hague: Martinus Nijhoff.

The Scottish Government (2008) Cabinet and ministers, biographies and responsibilities, http://www.scotland.gov.uk/About/14944/ Scottish- Cabinet.

Scotsman (2007) Danger from MRSA bugs supersedes bio-terrorism. 23 October 2007.

Selznick, P. (1949) *TVA and the Grass Roots: A Study in the Sociology of Formal Organization*. Berkeley, Calif.: University of California Press.

Sheaff, R. and Pilgrim, D. (2006) Can learning organizations survive in the newer NHS? *Implementation Science*. 1 (27): 1–11.

Shepherd, J. (2010) Goodbye Department for Curtains and Soft Furnishings: Gove renames DCSF the Department for Education as rainbow logos are taken down. *Guardian*, 13 May 2010, http://www.guardian.co.uk/education/2010/may/13/dcsf-new-name-department-education, accessed 14 April 2011.

Shipman Inquiry (2002) *First Report. Death Disguised*. London: HMSO, http://www.the-shipman-inquiry.org.uk/firstreport.asp, accessed 14 May 2010.

Shore, C. and Wright, S. (2000) Coercive accountability: the rise of audit culture in higher education. In *Audit Cultures: Anthropological Studies in Accountability, Ethics and Academy*, ed. M. Strathern. London: Routledge.

Simon, H. A. (1976) *Administrative Behavior: A Study of Decision-making Processes in Administrative Organization*. 2nd edition. London: Collier Macmillan.

Simon, H. (1982) *Models of Bounded Rationality*, Vol. I: *Economic Analysis and Public Policy*. Cambridge, Mass.: MIT Press.

Simon, H. (1986) Decision Making and Problem Solving. In *Research Briefings 1986: Report of the Research Briefing Panel on Decision Making and Problem Solving*. Washington, DC: National Academy Press, http://www. dieoff.org/page163.htm, accessed 24 November 2008.

Smith, G. and May, D. (1993) The artificial debate between rationalist and incrementalist models of decision making. In *The Policy Process: A Reader*, ed. M. Hill. New York: Harvester Wheatsheaf, pp. 197–211.

Smith, R. (1998) All changed, all changed utterly: British medicine will be transformed by the Bristol case. *BMJ*. 316: 1917–18.

Smith, R. (2000) The failings of NICE: time to start work on version 2. *BMJ*. 321: 1363–4.

Smith, R. (2005) Medical journals are an extension of the marketing arm of pharmaceutical companies. *PLoS Med.* 2 (5): e138.

Sparrow, A. (2001) Sept 11: 'a good day to bury bad news', http://www.telegraph.co.uk/news/uknews/1358985/Sept-11-a-good-day-to-bury-bad-news.html, accessed 8 April 2010.

Spector, M. and Kitsuse, J. (1987) *Constructing Social Problems.* New York: Aldine De Gruyter.

Spiegelhalter, D. J., Evans, S., Aylin, P. and Murray, G. (2000) *Overview of Statistical Evidence Presented to the Bristol Royal Infirmary Inquiry concerning the Nature and Outcomes of Paediatric Cardiac Surgical Services at Bristol relative to Other Specialist Centres from 1984 to 1995,* http://www.bristol-inquiry.org.uk/final_report/annex_b/images/Spiegelhalteretal_O_statev1.pdf, accessed 27 April 2010.

Sturgeon, N. (2007) Statement on abolition of prescription charges at the Scottish Parliament, Holyrood, Edinburgh, 5 December 2007, http://www.scotland.gov.uk/News/This-Week/Speeches/prescription-charges, accessed 26 November 2008.

Szmukler, G. (2000) Homicide inquiries: what sense do they make? *Psychiatrist* 24: 6–10, http://pb.rcpsych.org/cgi/content/full/24/1/6, accessed 13 May 2010.

Szmukler, G. and Holloway, F. (2001) *Mental Health Law: Discrimination or Protection?* Maudsley Discussion Papers, Paper 10, http://admin.iop.kcl.ac.uk/maudsley-publications/ maudsley-discussion-papers/mdp10.pdf, accessed 15 November 2004.

Taylor, P. and Gunn, J. (1999) Homicides by people with mental illness: myth and reality. *British Journal of Psychiatry.* 174: 9–14.

Taylor-Gooby, P. (2006) Trust, risk and health care reform. *Health, Risk and Society.* 8 (3): 1–7.

Taylor-Gooby, P. (2008) *Reframing Social Citizenship.* Oxford: Oxford University Press.

Thain, C. and Wright, M. (1995) *The Treasury and Whitehall: The Planning and Control of Public Expenditure, 1976–1993.* Oxford: Clarendon Press.

Tiefer, L. (2006) Female sexual dysfunction: a case study of disease mongering and active resistance. *PLoS Med.* 3 (4): e178.

Townsend, D. and Davidson, N. (1982) *Inequalities in Health: The Black Report.* London: Penguin Books.

Toynbee, P. (2010) The most perilous of cuts is to sever the historical record. *Guardian* 8 June 2010.

Tsebelis, G. (2002) *Veto Players: How Political Institutions Work.* Princeton: Princeton University Press.

Turner, B. A. and Pidgeon, N. E. (1997) *Man-Made Disasters.* 2nd edition. Oxford: Butterworth-Heinmann.

ushistory (n.d.) The Declaration of Independence, http://www.ushistory.org/declaration/document/, accessed 11 April 2011.

Vincent, C., Neale, G., and Woloshynowych, M. (2001) Adverse events in British hospitals: preliminary retrospective record review. *BMJ*. 322: 517–19.

Wakley, T. (1841) Editorial, *Lancet*, 1841–2 (2): 246.

Walt, G. (1994) *Health Policy: An Introduction to Process and Power*. London: Zed Books.

Wanless, D. (2002) *Securing our Future Health: Taking a Long-term View, Final Report*. London: Her Majesty's Treasury, http://www.hm-treasury. gov.uk/consult_wanless_final.htm, accessed 27 July 2009.

Warner, J. (2006) Inquiry reports as active texts and their function in relation to professional practice in mental health. *Health, Risk and Society*. 8: 223–37.

Washer, P. and Joffe, H. (2006) The hospital 'superbug': social representations of MRSA. *Social Science and Medicine*. 63 (8): 2141–52.

Webb, S. and Webb, B. (eds.) (1909) *The Break-up of the Poor Law: Being Part One of the Minority Report of the Poor Law Commission*. London: Longmans, Green and Co.

Weber, M. (1947) *The Theory of Social and Economic Organizations*. New York: Free Press of Glencoe.

Weber, M. (1968) *Economy and Society*, Vol. I. New York: Bedminster.

Weber, M. (2002) [1930] *The Protestant Ethic and the 'Spirit' of Capitalism, and Other Writings*. London: Penguin.

Webster, C. (1988) *The Health Services since the War*, Vol. I: *Problems of Health Care – The National Health Service before 1957*. London: HMSO.

Wheeler, M. (1997) *Politics and the Mass Media*. Oxford: Blackwell.

Woolgar, S. and Pawluch, D. (1985) Ontological gerrymandering: the anatomy of social problems explanations. *Social Problems*. 32 (3): 214–27.

Wright, T. and Evans, R. H. (1851) *Historical and descriptive account of the caricatures of James Gillray, comprising a political and humorous history of the latter part of the Reign of George the Third*. London: Henry G. Bohn, http://books.google.com/books?id=p_kjAAAAMAAJ&printsec=frontcov er&source=gbs_book_other_versions_r&cad=2_0#v=onepage&q=&f=fa lse, accessed 4 March 2010.

The Zito Trust (2009) *The Closure of the Zito Trust: Statement by the Trustees*, http:/www.zitotrust.co.uk, accessed 17 May 2010.

Žižek, S. (1989) *The Sublime Object of Ideology*. London: Verso.

Žižek, S. (1994) *Mapping Ideology*. London: Verso.

Index